Copyright

Copyright 2024. All rights reserved. No part of the material may be reproduced or utilized in any form without permission from the copyright owner.

The content, statements, views, and opinions herein are the sole expression of the authors. Reference to any specific commercial product, process, and service by trade name, trademark, manufacturer, or otherwise does not constitute or imply endorsement or recommendation. Gastroenterology Hospital Handbook is an independent publication and has not been authorized, sponsored, or approved by owners of the trademarks or services referenced in the book.

The authors have made every effort to provide accurate information. However, they are not responsible for efforts, omissions, or any outcomes related to the use of the contents of this book and take no responsibility for the use of the products or procedures described. Treatments and side effects described in this book may not apply to a patient. Drugs and medical devices discussed may have limited availability controlled by the Food and Drug Administration (FDA) for clinical use.

When considering a diagnostic test or treatment for an individual patient, the healthcare provider or reader is solely responsible for determining the needed testing and treatment plan. The healthcare provider or reader is also solely responsible for reviewing FDA status, reading package inserts, and reviewing prescribing information.

GASTROENTEROLOGY HOSPITAL HANDBOOK

VOLUME 2

A Practical Guide to Evaluation and Management

2024 Update

MARK PRINCE, MD

JULIANNA LINDSEY, MD

TABLE OF CONTENTS

1. Gastroenterology History
2. Gastroenterology Exam
3. Labs and Imaging
4. Endoscopy
5. Abdominal pain, epigastric and RUQ
6. Abdominal pain, RLQ and LLQ
7. Upper GI bleed, Hematemesis/Melena
8. Lower GI bleed, Hematochezia
9. Jaundice / Increased LFT
10. Ascites / Cirrhosis
11. Liver Failure
12. Pancreatitis / Increased Lipase
13. Inflammatory Bowel Disease
14. Dysphagia
15. Nausea / Vomiting
16. Diarrhea
17. Constipation / Ileus / PSBO
18. New Mass / Abnormal CT
19. Malnutrition / Enteral Tubes
20. GI surgeries

INTRODUCTION

Our handbook is designed to be a practical guide for the care of hospitalized patients with gastrointestinal complaints. We will focus on initial history, physical exam, and diagnostics.
Inpatient care is increasingly a team function. Multiple providers typically will evaluate a gastroenterology patient: initial evaluation in the emergency department, admission by hospitalists or intensivists, and gastroenterology consultation. Not all hospitals have GI resources immediately available. Our book is intended to be a valuable resource for mid-level providers, generalist physicians, and specialists.

Optimal care requires focus at each evaluation step, patient and provider communication, and efficient resource use. The wrong initial diagnosis and/or lack of communication can slow recovery and prolong hospital stays. Testing and therapies evolve, but the patient interview, examination, and plan development process remain constant. Key history, physical exam, and objective data relevant to gastroenterology will be outlined.

A cognitive decision framework is used to analyze acquired data to assist in development of differential diagnosis for common scenarios. After the initial differential diagnosis is constructed, appropriate testing can confirm and allow treatment to begin. We hope this handbook will be a resource and/or refresher for providers who evaluate GI patients.

1. GASTROENTEROLOGY HISTORY

Take-Aways:

- *Take your time. Getting an accurate description of the presenting complaint is critical.*
- *Introduce yourself and sit down. Sitting will improve patient trust and satisfaction.*
- *Correlate reported symptoms to eating, drinking, and bowel movements.*
- *Location is the most valuable descriptor of pain.*
- *Ask GI-specific review of systems questions.*

Obtaining an accurate history of presenting illness is the key to an efficient and effective evaluation. As Sir William Osler said, **"patients will tell you what is wrong with them if you will listen**." Understanding the narrative of each patient's illness is critical. After introducing yourself, sit down. Sitting down will help you gain trust with the patient and family.

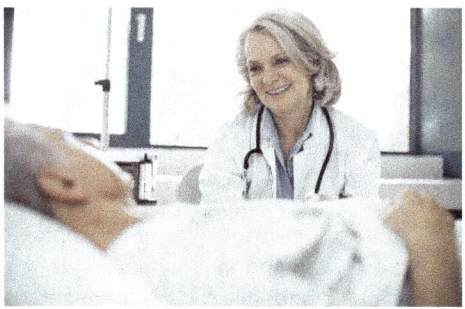

Ask the patient, family, and/or caregivers to restate the presenting symptoms. Do not rely on the recorded chief complaint in the medical record. Ask the patient yourself. Accurate information will save resources, shorten hospital stay, and get your patient well sooner.

Presenting details include the onset, location, duration, severity, quality, context, and associated symptoms. **Location** is usually the most helpful descriptor, especially with abdominal pain.

In addition, the **relationship** between food intake and bowel movements is important. Ask about the most recent oral intake in case an emergency procedure is necessary. Verbally "**read-back**" a symptom summary to increase patient confidence in you and allow for corrections.

All **medications**, including prescription, over-the-counter, and herbal supplements, are important. Anticoagulant and antiplatelet use must be considered before endoscopic or surgical procedures. New GLP-1 agonist medications can delay gastric emptying and require attention because delayed gastric emptying increases the risk of aspiration.

Previous medical and surgical history are needed to understand the current illness. **Weight loss surgery** is particularly important since the digestive anatomy can be altered. Frequently, gastroenterology inpatients are older and have comorbidities. With increasing obesity and obstructive sleep apnea, assess respiratory and overall functional status prior to scheduling procedures.

Behaviors like smoking, smokeless tobacco, EtOH, and illicit drugs are risk factors for many disorders. Ask about **marijuana use** in patients with nausea or vomiting. Do not assume elderly or "clean" patients do not use illicit drugs. In certain cases, travel, work, and environmental exposure can contribute to the presenting illness.

Medical records should always be reviewed for endoscopic procedures, pathology reports, and abdominal imaging. If radiology images are available, personally review them and correlate findings with the location of abdominal pain.

Ask about a **family history** of GI cancer or inflammatory bowel disease. Specific GI review of system questions includes weight loss, yellow or red eyes, cough while eating, nighttime diarrhea, the air in the urine stream, itching, and new insomnia or confusion.

In summary, personally asking the specifics of the presenting illness is critical to getting your patient on the correct diagnostic and therapeutic path. Spend a few minutes confirming the details *before* ordering tests which may or may not be needed. Treat the patient not the lab/imaging findings.

History:
HPI: location, severity, quality, context, association, duration
Past medical: medical, surgical, endoscopies, CT/MRI
Allergies: medications, foods, x-ray contrast
Medications: prescription, over the counter, supplements
Social: tobacco, EtOH, illicit drugs, work and travel history
Family: GI cancers, chronic pancreatitis, Crohn's/ulcerative colitis

Review of systems:
Constitutional: weight loss, fever
Eyes: red eyes, yellow eyes
Ear, nose, throat: mouth sores, pain on swallowing
Respiratory: cough when eating, cough with sleeping/lying flat
Cardiovascular: chest pain with swallowing, LE edema
Gastrointestinal: heartburn, difficulty swallowing, nausea, vomiting, pain, constipation, diarrhea, bleeding
Genitourinary: blood in urine, air in urine
Musculoskeletal: joint/back pain
Skin: yellow skin, itching, redness of palms
Neurological: tremor, change in speech pattern
Psychiatric: insomnia, confusion
Endocrine: night sweats, flushing
Hematologic: swollen nodes, fatigue
Allergy: food allergies and sensitivity (lactose, gluten)

2. GASTROENTEROLOGY EXAM

Take-Aways:

- *Begin your evaluation with initial vital signs and estimate the patient's overall level of distress.*
- *Baseline vital signs help estimate volume status/ fluid loss and can signal patient toxicity.*
- *Divide the abdominal exam into four quadrants and correlate exam findings with the underlying anatomy.*
- *Examine skin for signs of liver or inflammatory bowel disease. Liver disease may cause tremor or confusion.*
- *Atypical findings may occur in the elderly or immunosuppressed.*

Begin your evaluation with vital signs, patients with significant **dehydration** and/or **bleeding** need volume deficits corrected. The amount of fluid loss can be estimated by the physical exam.[1] Blood pressure, pulse, respiratory rate, skin, and mental status will help to estimate blood loss.[2]

Volume Loss	Systolic BP	Pulse	Respirations	Skin	Mentation
10-15%	nl	nl	nl	nl	nl
15-30%	nl	>100	>15	pale	restless
30-40%	<100	>120	>20	clammy	confused
>40%	<70	>140	>30	cool	lethargic

The inability to mount an effective inflammatory response (and lack of elevated temperature) may occur in **cirrhosis** or **sepsis**. Height and weight are useful to calculate body mass index (**BMI**). Obesity is a risk factor for GI illness and a significant risk for sedated procedures or surgeries. However, a low BMI should prompt a nutritional evaluation. Continuing with patient observation, look for restlessness, obvious pain, and overall level of hygiene. Be concerned for intestinal ischemia when reported pain is worse than objective physical exam findings.

Examine the eyes, mouth, and skin for signs of liver or inflammatory bowel disease. Jaundice, icterus, spider angiomata, and palmar erythema may indicate underlying liver disease.

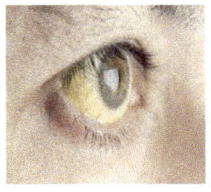 Icterus 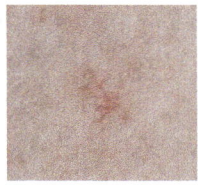 angiomata

Look directly at the abdomen for surgical scars and abdominal hernia (hernias are frequently near the umbilicus and groin). Palpate for masses and estimate if abdominal pain is from superficial structures or from a deeper source. Abdominal guarding with palpation or rigidity suggests **peritonitis** (inflammation/perforation). Dullness to percussion can be related to intra-abdominal fluid **(ascites)**. Finally, auscultation allows the assessment of bowel sounds. High-pitched bowel sounds suggest a **bowel obstruction**. A rectal exam is mandatory for any patient with rectal or perineal pain. After your examination, correlate findings with the underlying intra-abdominal anatomy.

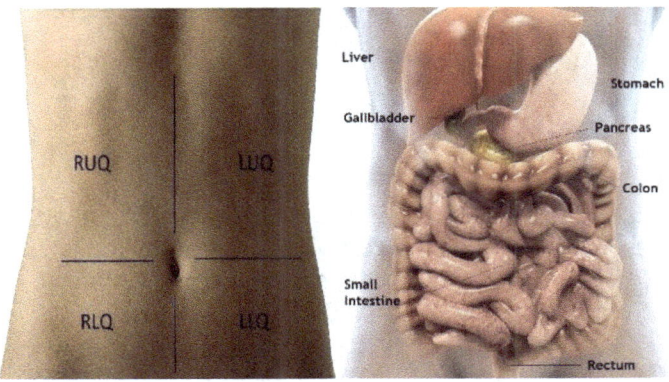

Females with **pelvic pain** should have a pelvic exam performed prior to admission in the emergency department. A **bimanual exam** can be performed at the bedside (remember to have a chaperone regardless of the examiner's gender).

Not all abdominal pain is from an intraabdominal source. Pain can be related to rib margin inflammation, rectus abdominal muscle pain, or disorders of the skin (zoster). Again, examination through a gown is not adequate. Look directly at the skin. Specific maneuvers or findings such as **Carnett's sign** (abdominal wall pain), **Murphy's sign** (gallbladder), and **Grey Turner's sign** (pancreatitis) can suggest an underlying etiology. Examination may have atypical or unreliable findings in the elderly or immunosuppressed.[3]

Notes:

Carnett's sign: ask the patient to point with one finger to where it hurts, then apply pressure to the painful spot. Ask the patient to either sit up or raise both legs above the table at the same time. Patients with abdominal wall pain will have an increase in pain, whereas patients with an internal source of pain may have a decrease in pain.

Murphy's sign: pain on palpation of the RUQ beneath the costal margin, classically worse with inspiration.

Cullen's sign: edema/bruising around the umbilicus

Grey/Turner's sign: bruising of the flank

Physical exam:

Vitals: BP, pulse, respirations, temperature, height, weight, O_2 sat
General: overall appearance, level of hygiene
Eyes: pale conjunctiva, icterus, episcleritis, xanthelasma
ENT: oral ulcers, state of dentition, oral thrush
Neck: thyromegaly, neck masses
Chest: respiratory effort, rate, lung sounds
CV: heart rate, LE edema
Abd: scars, hernias, bowel sounds, tenderness, distention, hepatomegaly, rectal exam findings

Skin: jaundice, angiomata, rashes (e. nodosum or pyoderma)
Neuro: alertness, tremors, asterixis
MS: joint inflammation, joint deformity
Lymphatic: infraclavicular adenopathy (Virchow's node), periumbilical adenopathy (Sister Mary Joseph's node)
Psych: psychomotor slowing, confusion, intoxication

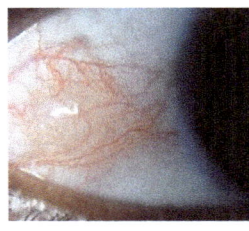 Episcleritis

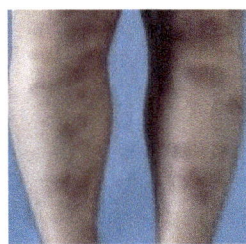 Erythema nodosum

3. LABS AND IMAGING

Take-Aways:

- *BMP, CBC, LFT, Lipase, UA, and urine pregnancy are basic labs and add Pt/INR for all liver disease patients.*
- *Initial HGB/HCT may underestimate the amount of blood loss with GI bleeding.*
- *Liver testing requires a balance for needed but not excessive lab evaluation.*
- *Ultrasound is the initial imaging modality for liver and gallbladder evaluation.*
- *Multidetector CT scan is the best overall abdominal imaging. IV contrast will enhance visualization.*

Basic **abdominal pain** labs include a CBC, BMP, LFT, lipase, UA, urine pregnancy test (age-appropriate females) and Pt/INR. **Liver disease** evaluation can include ammonia level, ANA, acute hepatitis panel, Fe/TIBC, acetaminophen level, Etoh level, urine drug screen. Exhaustive testing including smooth muscle antibody, anti-liver kidney microsomal antibody, ceruloplasmin, alpha-one antitrypsin, hereditary hemochromatosis, and liver fibrosis are generally unnecessary for inpatient evaluation. Esoteric (and expensive) tests can be obtained in outpatient follow up. With increasing costs in healthcare, **resource utilization** is a consideration. Getting extensive labs is usually not helpful, but always increases cost.

When **pancreatic disease** occurs, lipase is needed. If diarrhea occurs with pancreatic disease, stool fat and stool elastase can be helpful estimating pancreatic insufficiency. Inflammatory bowel disease (IBD) labs include ESR, CRP, stool studies for WBC, culture, O+P, and C. diff. Other testing like stool calprotectin, ASCA, ANCA, and IBD panels are not needed for initial evaluation.

Tumor marker labs like alpha-feto protein, CEA, CA 19-9, and CA 125 are not diagnostic of cancer. Tumor markers can be useful to oncologists to help guide workup when a mass is found on imaging. Remember that tumor markers can be increased in benign or inflammatory conditions.

An increased tumor marker frequently leads to confusion, increased imaging, and delayed hospital discharge during inpatient evaluation. If there is no obvious mass, avoid ordering tumor markers. Even when a mass is found, a biopsy is needed. **Tumor markers are no substitute for a tissue biopsy.**

Common imaging for inpatients are plain abdominal X-rays, abdominal ultrasound, and a multidetector CT scan. Biliary imaging can be performed with magnetic retrograde cholangiopancreatography (MRCP). Plain abdominal X-rays can define the interface between bowel gas and fluid in the digestive tract. Conditions like perforation, ileus, and bowel obstruction will have bowel gas irregularities.

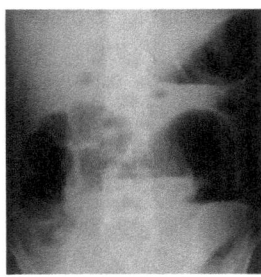 X-ray: air-fluid levels

Ultrasound is particularly effective when the ultrasound transducer is close to the target organ (like the liver and gallbladder). Liver masses, fatty liver, thickened gallbladder wall, and gallstones can be found on RUQ ultrasound.

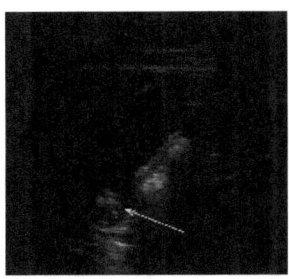 Ultrasound: gallbladder stone

Liver blood flow abnormalities can be evaluated with **hepatic doppler**. Doppler can be done simultaneously with a RUQ ultrasound. Normal blood flow in the portal vein is towards the liver (termed hepatotedal flow). Abnormal blood flow is away from the portal vein (termed hepatofugal flow). Hepatofugal flow is caused by a variety of liver diseases such as advanced cirrhosis.

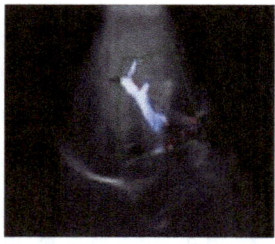 Liver doppler: hepatofugal flow

CT imaging is the best overall view of the abdomen/pelvis. Advanced image formating allows for excellent views in both axial and coronal imaging. The addition of oral and IV contrast will improve definition of the vascular and digestive structures. Gallstones, intestinal inflammation, abdominal masses, and non digestive abnormalities can be evaluated with CT imaging.

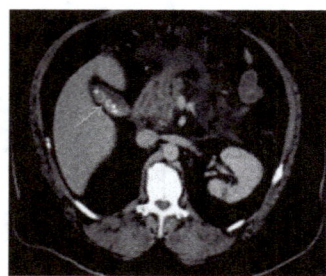 CT: gallstones

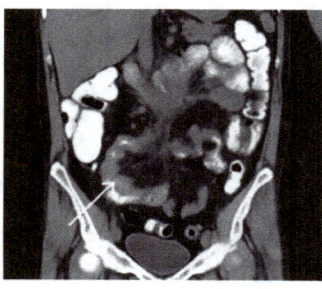 CT coronal view: ileitis

CT angiography (CTA) is particularly useful for brisk lower GI bleeding. With significant bleeding, contrast extravasation will mirror the site of bleeding. CT angiography done in the emergency department can estimate the bleeding source and guide further treatment.

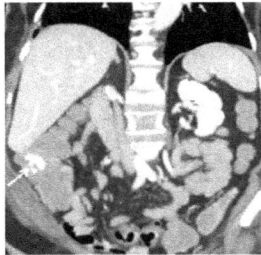
CTA: contrast extravasation

MRI and MRCP can add additional information regarding the biliary tree and pancreas. MRI, with or without contrast, can refine possible anomalies found on other imaging. MRCP is non-contrast imaging and can provide detailed images of the common bile duct and pancreatic duct. If an ERCP is planned, a MRCP is not always needed. Again, consider resource utilization.

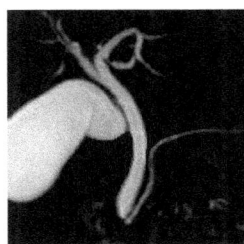
MRCP: normal anatomy

Nuclear medicine imaging includes nuclear medicine bleeding scan and HIDA scan to evaluate the patency of the cystic duct and exclude acute cholecystitis. HIDA can also be performed with an evaluation of the gallbladder ejection fraction to evaluate for poor gallbladder emptying (biliary dyskinesia).

Modified barium swallow is the preferred imaging for oropharyngeal dysphagia and to evaluate for aspiration. Tests rarely ordered on inpatients include gastric emptying scan, octreotide scan, liver elastography, upper GI series, barium enema, and barium defecography.

Interventional radiology (IR) procedures allow for diagnostic and therapeutic interventions. Biopsy of mass/tumors needing inpatient diagnosis can be performed. Embolization of bleeding sources, empiric embolization of gastroduodenal artery for recurrent bleeding, TIPS for portal hypertension, and placement of drains for abscess/fluid collections are common procedures. Interventional radiology procedures are less invasive than surgery.

When you are unsure which imaging modality to order, **call your radiologist.** A quick phone call can prevent unnecessary testing and wasted time and resources.

4. ENDOSCOPY

Take-Aways:

- *Endoscopy is the foundation of modern gastroenterology.*
- *Key question: "Is my patient healthy enough to be sedated for a GI procedure?"*
- *Except for a true emergency, patients must be NPO prior to an endoscopic procedure.*
- *A good colon prep is important for colonoscopy.*
- *ERCP and EUS are increasingly therapeutic procedures.*

Endoscopy is the cornerstone of gastroenterology and has revolutionized the diagnosis and treatment of digestive disorders over the last 50 years. The ability to visualize the mucosa, get a sample for laboratory/pathology, and perform ever-expanding therapeutic interventions is central to gastroenterology.

"Is my patient healthy enough to undergo sedation/anesthesia?" is critical. Inpatients are frequently ill and will undergo scrutiny of your anesthesia service prior to sedation. Propofol anesthesia carries the same perioperative cardiovascular risk as general anesthesia. Depending upon the length of the procedure and your local anesthesiology practices, routine endotracheal intubation may occur for procedures like foreign body removal, ERCP, EUS, and device-assisted enteroscopy.

Coagulopathy or medications that promote bleeding should be addressed prior to endoscopy. Except for emergency procedures, patients must be **NPO** 2-3 hours after clear liquids, 4-6 hours after full liquids, or 7-8 hours after any food intake to minimize aspiration of gastric contents.

EGD (esophagogastroduodenoscopy) is the visual assessment of the esophagus, stomach, and duodenum. Sampling of the gastric mucosa for H. pylori infection can be taken. EGD is the most frequent inpatient endoscopic procedure.

Common indications are GI bleeding, upper abdominal pain, difficulty swallowing, nausea/vomiting, and placement of an enteral feeding tube. Esophagitis, gastritis, and gastroduodenal ulcers are frequent findings.

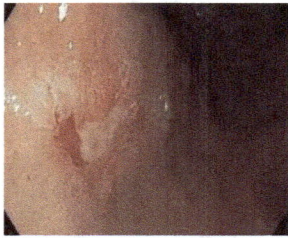 EGD: bleeding gastric ulcer

Colonoscopy is the visual assessment of the colon and, occasionally, the terminal ileum. Laxative preparation is required to flush colon contents out to allow for mucosal visualization. Preparation usually involves an oral laxative like golytely, miralax, or bisacodyl. When oral preparation is impossible, a combination of suppositories and enemas can be used, but the preparation will likely be poor. Common indications for colonoscopy are GI bleeding, lower abdominal pain, diarrhea, and abnormal CT scan. Diverticulosis, colon polyps/tumors, Crohn's ulceration, and ulcerative colitis are possible.

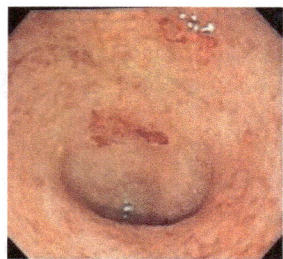 Colonoscopy: ulcerative colitis

Capsule endoscopy is used to evaluate the small intestine by swallowing a disposable capsule containing a camera, battery, and image transmitter. The capsule records 8-12 hours of images which are downloaded to a workstation. Common indication for capsule endoscopy is obscure GI bleeding Take note that capsule endoscopy is usually contraindicated in patients at risk of bowel obstruction (fear of capsule retention requiring surgical removal)

and for patients with a pacemaker. Capsule endoscopy is only a diagnostic exam (no therapeutic options) and does require time for imaging, download, and physician review. Delay in hospital discharge can occur. Therefore, in stable patients, capsule endoscopy frequently is scheduled as an outpatient procedure.

ERCP (endoscopic retrograde cholangiopancreatography) is performed with a side viewing duodenoscope and fluoroscopic imaging of the bile and/or pancreatic ducts. ERCP reveals excellent images of the duodenal wall where the major and minor papilla are located. Fluoroscopy assists in the diagnosis and treatment of biliary tract stones, strictures, bile leaks, and pancreatic disorders. Common reasons for inpatient ERCP are suspected bile duct stones, jaundice, and biliary stent placement. ERCP is the most dangerous GI procedure performed. The risk of **post-ERCP pancreatitis** is approximately 5%.

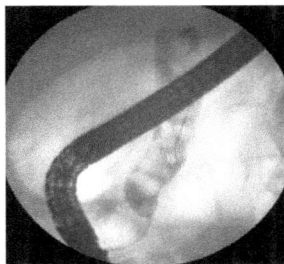 ERCP: biliary stones

EUS (endoscopic ultrasound) combines visual assessment of the GI mucosa with ultrasound imaging of the digestive tract wall and/or surrounding structures. Initially a diagnostic test, the use of endoscopic ultrasound-guided fine needle biopsy, fine needle injection, and drainage of abdominal fluid collections has expanded interventional applications. Common reasons for an inpatient EUS are pancreatic mass evaluation and drainage of fluid collections (pancreatic pseudocyst or rectal abscess).

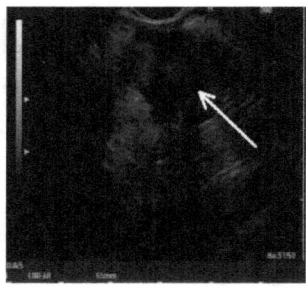 EUS: pancreatic mass

SBE (small bowel enteroscopy) provides a visual assessment of the jejunum and/or ileum. SBE, in simple terms, is an extended EGD done from above or an extended colonoscopy from below using a longer scope. Specialized enteroscopes and device-assisted systems like single or double balloon enteroscopy allow for visualizing more of the small bowel. Common inpatient reasons for a small bowel enteroscopy are GI bleeding, abnormal capsule endoscopy, or abnormal CT scan. Given the therapeutic possibilities, SBE is frequently done in cases of obscure GI bleeding (instead of an inpatient capsule endoscopy).

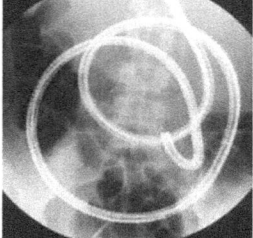 Fluoroscopy: enteroscope

Other GI procedures, such as esophageal motility, acid reflux testing, liver elastography, breath hydrogen testing, and anorectal motility, are rarely performed on inpatients.

5. ABDOMINAL PAIN: Epigastric / Right Upper Quadrant

Take-Aways:

- *Location is a helpful descriptor for pain. Correlate location of pain with underlying abdominal anatomy.*
- *Peptic ulcer and biliary disease are common causes.*
- *H. pylori antibody testing (IgG) does not indicate acute infection. Do not order H. pylori antibody for inpatients.*
- *Ultrasound is excellent imaging for the gallbladder, but CT imaging is better overall for the upper abdomen.*
- *PPIs are overused. BID PPI is rarely needed for inpatients. Histamine$_2$ blockers can be an acceptable alternative.*

Upper abdominal pain is a strong motivator for patients to come to the hospital. The differential diagnosis of upper abdominal pain is vast and includes non-digestive pain. **Peptic ulcer** and **gallbladder disease** are the most common causes of upper abdominal pain. Symptom location is the most important clue, and relating underlying abdominal anatomy to the location of pain will help you develop a differential diagnosis.

The peritoneal surface can be irritated causing localized pain. However, diffuse or referred pain can be present from **non-digestive causes** such as right lower lobe pneumonia, cardiac pain, abdominal wall pain, and pyelonephritis. The **Onset** and **severity** of pain are important. **Rapid** onset of **severe** pain suggests active inflammation. Whereas **mild to moderate** severity is suggestive of visceral pain. Increasing pain with movement, external pressure, or cough suggests peritoneal inflammation. Food intake may worsen the pain of a gastric ulcer, but eating might reduce the pain of a duodenal ulcer. Any food intake can worsen gallbladder pain. Take note of anticoagulants, NSAIDs, smoking, Etoh, and GI surgeries.

The **abdominal exam** is vital to identify the need for urgent intervention. Begin with resting vital signs; persistent tachycardia or tachypnea are worrisome. Do not ignore the initial vital signs! A **restless patient** is suggestive of gallbladder disease or pancreatitis. A patient lying **very still** and avoiding movement may have peritonitis. **Look directly** at the skin for scars, hernias, or discoloration. The abdominal skin should be exposed for your exam. Begin away from the site of pain. If the abdomen is hard or seems to have a persistent muscle spasm, rigidity is present. Next, **palpate** for enlargement of the liver or spleen, and exam for ascites (dullness to percussion or bulging flanks).

Labs include CBC, BMP, LFT, lipase, urinalysis, urine pregnancy test (age-appropriate females). Imaging frequently includes an abdominal ultrasound and/or CT scan. **Ultrasound** is especially beneficial for conditions located near the skin and is the test of choice for RUQ pain or suspected gallstones.

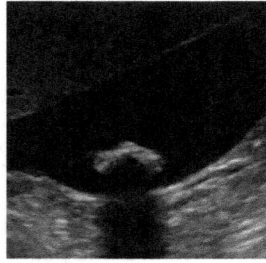 Ultrasound: stone with shadow

Ultrasound is best done in the fasting state, as the gallbladder contracts after eating, reducing visualization. Gallstones, biliary sludge, wall inflammation, or pericholecystic fluid suggest a **gallbladder source** of pain.

Computed tomography **(CT)** has become the preferred imaging modality for abdominal pain. IV (intravenous) and oral contrast increase the visibility of the digestive tract and solid organs. In cases where biliary disease is suspected but not definite, **MRCP** can provide excellent imaging of the bile and pancreatic ducts.

Disease	Location	Association	Referred Pain
esophagitis	epigastric	dysphagia	chest
gastritis/PUD	epigastric	belching	RUQ
cholecystitis	RUQ	nausea	right shoulder
hepatitis	RUQ	jaundice	right shoulder
pancreatitis	epigastric	vomiting	back

The common cause of esophagitis is **gastroesophageal reflux**. The retrograde flow of gastric liquids can result in pain and mucosal damage. Risk factors for reflux esophagitis include intermittent lower esophageal sphincter relaxation and a hiatal hernia. As society develops higher rates of obesity, more patients are developing GERD.[4]

EGD is the test of choice for heartburn and epigastric pain. Tests such as barium esophagogram or esophageal motility are not suggested for inpatient evaluation. The mainstay for GERD treatment is lifestyle modification with reduction of caffeine, peppermints, smoking, and EtOH. Once daily PPI is the most prescribed medication, but potential side effects are of increasing concern. BID or high-dose PPI therapy is discouraged. Other causes of esophagitis include infections (candidiasis, CMV, HSV), pill esophagitis (potassium, doxycycline, alendronate), and radiation esophagitis.

Irritation and/or inflammation of gastric mucosa occurs when the protective mucus layer is impaired. Peptic ulcer disease **(PUD)** can occur. **Common causes** of PUD are H. pylori and NSAID use. H. pylori is a gram-negative bacterium that weakens the gastric mucus layer. Eventually, ulceration into the gastric submucosa can occur.

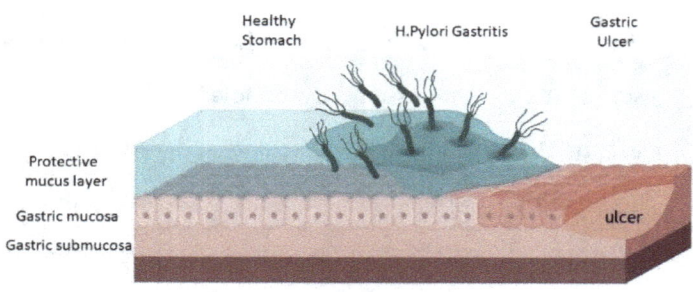

H.Pylori Induced Gastric Ulcer

H. pylori is a risk factor for gastric adenocarcinoma. Testing is usually done with endoscopic biopsy for pathology. Stool antigen testing for H. pylori can evaluate for an acute infection. H. pylori blood serology (IgG) measures antibody formation and is not confirmative of an acute infection. The utility of serologic testing is questionable. Therefore, serologic testing for H. pylori is not suggested in the hospital.

NSAIDs inhibit cyclooxygenase, reducing prostaglandins (important to maintaining the gastric mucus layer). **Enteric-coated, rectal, and oral NSAIDs** can all lead to PUD via systemic absorption and prostaglandin reduction of the gastric mucus layer. NSAIDs are worrisome in the elderly and patients taking prednisone. Cigarette smoking may interact with H. pylori to promote ulcer development and will impair ulcer healing.[5] Patients with serious illness (severe burns, head injury, and ICU stay) can develop gastric "**stress ulcers**".

EGD's key advantages are the ability to directly visualize the gastric mucosa, stop bleeding, and get biopsy samples. **PPI or H_2 blockers** are the most effective treatment medications for gastric ulcers. H_2 blockers work at the histamine site on gastric cells by competitive inhibition, reducing gastric acid production for 4-6 hours. BID dosing is needed to maintain effective acid suppression. PPIs reduce acid by binding the HK-ATPase on the gastric cell, reducing gastric acid production for 18-22 hours. Therefore, once-daily dosing is possible. Both H_2 and PPI are available in IV formulation. For most gastric ulcers, once daily, oral or IV PPI will promote ulcer healing.

For PUD with an elevated risk of rebleeding after endoscopic treatment, a 72-hour PPI infusion is particularly effective in reducing rebleeding risk. PPIs have become the mainstay for PUD because of the simplicity and once-a-day dosing. Rarely, gastric ulcers can be malignant. When a gastric ulcer is found and treated, a repeat EGD is suggested in 8-12 weeks to confirm ulcer healing. A non-healing ulcer should be biopsied and followed to exclude malignancy.

Cholecystitis is usually related to gallstones, which cause obstruction of the cystic duct. When the cystic duct is blocked, inflammation of the gallbladder occurs, resulting in severe pain.

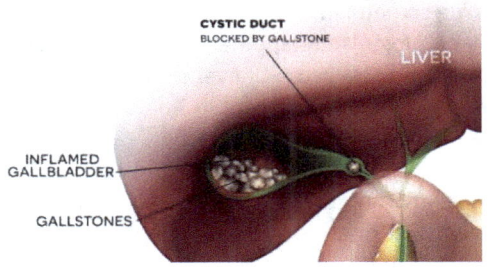

Murphy's sign- increased pain during palpation of the RUQ, which is worse on inspiration, is a classic sign of cholecystitis and was described by prominent Chicago surgeon Dr. John Murphy circa 1900. **Atypical symptoms** like right shoulder pain or nausea may lead to confusion regarding the diagnosis. Cholecystectomy is needed with cholecystitis. Risk factors for gallstones include female sex, increasing age, obesity, rapid weight loss, and Hispanic or Native American ethnicity.[6]

Passage of a gallstone into the common bile duct can cause significantly increased LFTs. Increases in bilirubin and/or alkaline phosphatase (especially with common bile duct dilation) suggests a bile duct stone. ERCP can confirm and remove stones before or after cholecystectomy. HIDA scan imaging can confirm if the cystic duct is patent or obstructed if cholecystitis is suspected but not confirmed. HIDA scan uses a radioactive tracer to follow the flow of bile. The cystic duct is not obstructed if the radiotracer is visualized in the gallbladder.

Acute hepatitis is swelling of the liver with stretching of the liver capsule. RUQ pain, nausea, malaise, and anorexia can occur. Viruses, EtOH, and medications are common etiologies. Question patients regarding over-the-counter supplement use, illicit drugs, travel, sexual activity, new piercings or tattoos, and sick contacts. On exam icterus, jaundice, mild hepatosplenomegaly, and RUQ pain with palpation may be present.

Hepatocellular injury with elevation of AST/ALT is the predominant laboratory finding. Ultrasound will usually be normal except for occasional hepatomegaly. Testing should include an acute viral hepatitis panel, ANA, Pt/INR, acetaminophen and EtOH levels, and urine drug screen . In selected patients, monospot, EBV serology, CMV serology, and hepatitis E antigen may be obtained. Pt/INR is a useful measure of liver synthetic function. **Supportive treatment** with monitoring of INR and for mental status changes are needed.

Acute pancreatitis is inflammation of the pancreas caused by pancreatic autodigestion from intrinsic enzymes. Given the location of the pancreas in the posterior upper abdomen, epigastric pain with radiation to the back is frequently reported.

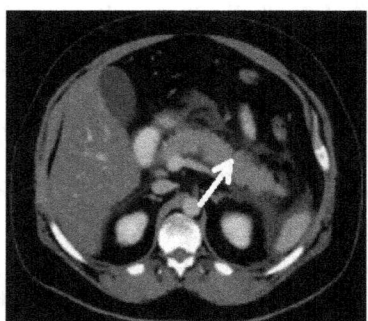
CT: acute pancreatitis

Pancreatitis patients will often find **relief sitting up** and leaning forward (as do patients with pericarditis). **Elevated lipase** (at least three times normal) and/or pancreatic inflammation on CT in patients with upper abdominal pain are needed to diagnose acute pancreatitis. Common etiologies include gallstones, biliary sludge, EtOH intake, hypercalcemia, and high triglycerides. Treatment is bowel rest, pain control, IV hydration, and supportive care. Initial IV fluids are critical in the first 24-36 hours to maintain excellent blood flow to the inflamed pancreas.

6. ABDOMINAL PAIN, LLQ / RLQ

Take-Aways:

- *Causes of lower abdominal pain include gastrointestinal, genitourinary, and post-surgical causes.*
- *Diverticulitis and colitis are common GI sources of pain.*
- *Physical exam is critical to evaluate for a "surgical abdomen." If doubt, get a surgical consultation.*
- *CT is the most instructive imaging modality.*

The differential diagnosis of lower abdominal pain is complicated by the pelvic anatomy and associated genitourinary organs. It is critical to understand the underlying abdominal anatomy when correlating pain location with potential causes. **Diverticulitis, infectious colitis,** and **ischemic colitis** are common colonic causes of pain. Non-digestive sources of lower abdominal pain include ovarian cysts, cystitis, pyelonephritis, kidney stones, and pelvic inflammatory disease.

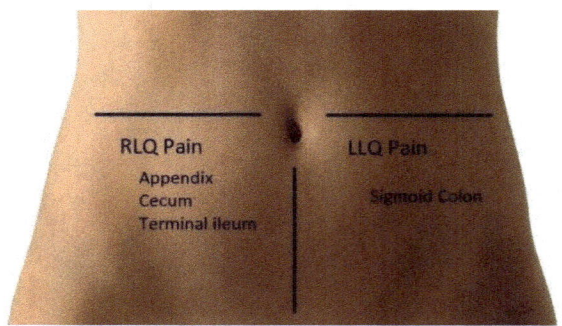

Increasing pain with movement, external pressure, or cough suggests peritoneal inflammation **(peritonitis).** Peritonitis causes include bowel perforation, ruptured abdominal aortic aneurysm, and severe intra-abdominal infection. In contrast, restless patients with lower abdominal/pelvic pain suggests a kidney stone or urinary tract infection.

The relationship of pain to urination, bowel movements, and sexual intercourse is valuable. Important **historical factors** are GI surgeries, last menstrual period, tampon usage, and last bowel movement.

Look directly at the skin, auscultate, and apply gentle pressure with your stethoscope. If involuntary abdominal muscle spasm occurs with pressure, **guarding** is present and suggests peritonitis. The rigidity of the abdominal muscles suggests a "surgical abdomen." **Ascites** may result in bulging of the flanks and/or shifting dullness to percussion. Groin and periumbilical exams may reveal hernias. Finally, a scrotal exam for men, pelvic exam for females, and digital rectal exam for all are needed with lower abdominal pain.

Labs for low abdominal pain includes CBC, BMP, LFT, urinalysis, and urine pregnancy test (age-appropriate females). Stool studies are necessary for diarrheal illness, including testing for culture, O+P, and C. diff. In addition, inflammatory markers like c-reactive protein or ESR are useful as a baseline measurement if an inflammatory process is suspected.

Ultrasound evaluates issues like appendicitis. Pelvic and transvaginal ultrasound can evaluate the female reproductive system. **CT imaging** is the most valuable modality and is an especially useful tool for acute surgical problems.

Disease	Location	Timing	Association	Referred Pain
Diverticulitis	LLQ	acute	fever	left flank
Colitis	RLQ/LLQ	acute/chronic	diarrhea	flanks
Ileitis	RLQ	acute/chronic	diarrhea	periumbilical
Appendicitis	RLQ	acute	fever	periumbilical
Hernia	RLQ/LLQ	acute/chronic	vomiting	scrotum

Diverticulitis is an infection within a diverticular pouch. Increasing colonic pressure can lead to formation of diverticular pouches. The sigmoid colon is the smallest diameter segment of the colon and, as such, has the potential for the highest internal pressure; therefore, the sigmoid colon is the most common site for diverticulosis and diverticulitis. Patients often complain of LLQ pain and reduced bowel movements; fever may also be present. An important clue for diverticulitis is the lack of significant bleeding. Labs frequently reveal an increased WBC. CT will show colon wall thickening in areas of diverticulosis. Rarely, an abscess will form extra-luminally or even perforate resulting in peritonitis.

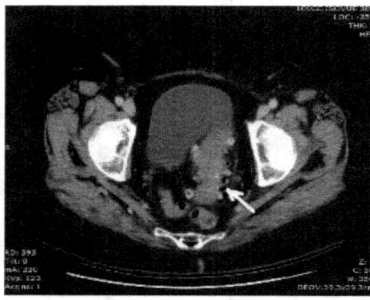
CT: sigmoid diverticulitis

Diverticulitis treatment is IV fluids and antibiotics. Acute diverticulitis is a contraindication to colonoscopy. However, a colonoscopy should be planned in 4-6 weeks after finishing antibiotics if a recent colonoscopy has not been performed to exclude colon cancer.

Acute infection is the most common cause of **colitis.** Other causes, such as Crohn's disease, ulcerative colitis, and ischemic colitis, are possible. Diarrhea with or without bleeding can occur. Inflammatory parameters like CRP and ESR can be elevated. **Stool testing** for culture, ova and parasites, and C. diff should be done on admission. If hematochezia and pain are present, **ischemic colitis** should be considered. Antibiotics can be given after stool collection. Consider colonoscopy to evaluate the colonic mucosa and obtain tissue biopsy samples if symptoms do not improve.

Ileitis is intestinal inflammation; the most common location for Crohn's disease is the terminal ileum. Symptoms include RLQ, hematochezia, and diarrhea. Unless signs of small bowel obstruction are present, a **colonoscopy** is needed to obtain a biopsy to evaluate for infection vs inflammatory bowel disease.

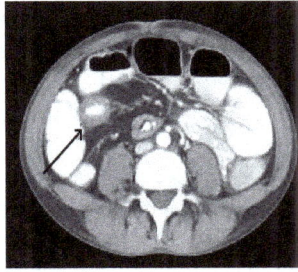
CT: RLQ ileal inflammation/ileitis

Appendicitis is the classic cause of RLQ pain especially in younger adults. The appendix is located at the base of the cecum with a diverticular type pouch. The opening is exposed to stool and contents of the cecum. When obstruction or inflammation of the appendix occurs, pain develops. Initially, the pain is more visceral and localized in the periumbilical area. Increasing inflammation will irritate the peritoneum, and pain localizes in the RLQ at McBurney's point (1/3 the distance from the anterior superior iliac spine to the umbilicus).

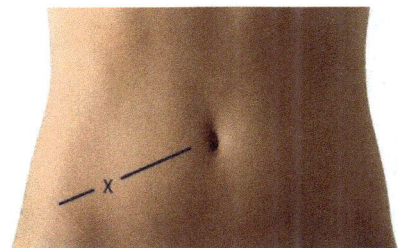
McBurney's point

Labs reveal a mild increase in WBC unless perforation has occurred, and imaging with either **RLQ ultrasound** or **CT** confirms the diagnosis. Imaging is suggested when acute appendicitis is suspected since up to **1/3 of patients will have an alternate diagnosis** after imaging results.[7] CT findings of a thickened wall, peri appendiceal fat stranding, and/or an appendicolith are suggestive of acute appendicitis.

Appendicitis is usually diagnosed in the emergency department, antibiotics are given, and a surgical consultation occurs. Treatment is surgical removal since an inflamed appendix can perforate and cause peritonitis. The risk of perforation is highest in the first 24-36 hours. Since the tip of the appendix can move, and symptoms can be atypical, keep appendicitis in the differential diagnosis of any unexplained right-sided **abdominal pain**.

Abdominal hernias are common in the inguinal canal and near the umbilicus. A swelling "bulge" with lifting, coughing, or movement suggest a hernia. Swelling will resolve with lying flat. **Two types** of inguinal hernia exist. **Direct hernias** develop medial to the vessels going through fascial weakness of the inguinal canal. **Indirect hernias** develop with protrusion through the deep inguinal ring on the descending path to the scrotum. Hernias are more common in men.

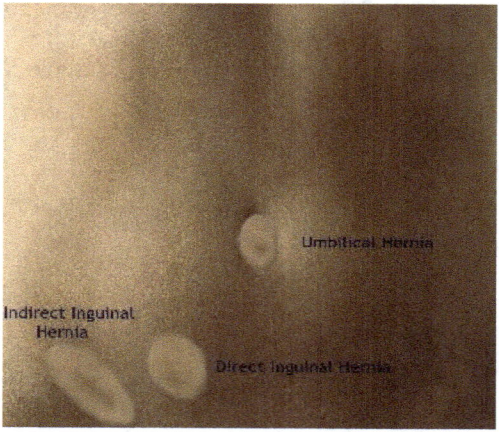

If abdominal contents become **entrapped** and cannot be reduced, incarceration can develop and progress to strangulation with ischemia and the potential for gangrene. Hernias are best examined with a patient standing with and without a cough. To **reduce a hernia**, the patient needs to be supine. If hernia cannot be reduced, urgent surgical consultation is needed.

7. UPPER GI BLEED, Hematemesis / Melena

Take-Aways:

- *Upper GI bleeding is dangerous with a high mortality.*
- *Hemodynamics and IV fluid resuscitation are critical.*
- *IV PPI, at least one dose, should be given initially on hospital presentation.*
- *EGD can diagnose, apply treatment, and determine prognosis.*

Upper GI bleeding is dangerous. Despite improved therapies, upper GI bleeding still has a **high mortality of 5-10%.**[8] Typically, **hematemesis** and **melena (black/tarry stools)** originate from a bleeding source in the esophagus, stomach, or duodenum. Carefully ask for a specific description of the color and severity of bleeding. Consider other sources of bleeding like hemoptysis and nosebleeds. With increasing age in the United States, associated cardiovascular comorbidities, anticoagulants, and antiplatelet use increase, and more GI bleeding is occurring. An accurate medication list is important. In addition, knowledge of the patient's use of OTC meds like NSAIDs and aspirin products is critical. The timing of the last meal is important when an urgent endoscopy may be needed.

The **resting BP and pulse** are instructive to the severity of bleeding. Dry oral mucosa, poor capillary refill, tachycardia, and orthostatic hypotension are signs of **volume depletion**. Physical exam stigmata of cirrhosis and/or ascites should be noted as prophylactic antibiotics are needed for cirrhotic patients prior to upper endoscopy to minimize the potential for spontaneous bacterial peritonitis.

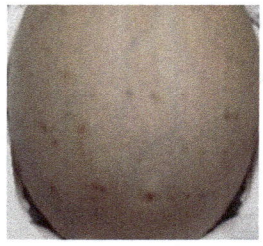
Ascites

NG tube lavage of the stomach can determine the color and amount of bleeding. Red blood in vomitus and/or NG lavage suggests urgent endoscopy is needed. Patients bleed whole blood (RBC and plasma). Therefore, **the initial hematocrit (HCT) may be normal**. However, with the replacement of IV fluids, the HCT will drop. GI bleeding increases nitrogen load in the gut, and an **elevated BUN** is frequently seen. Measure the Pt/INR, CBC, and BMP. Unless perforation is suspected, abdominal imaging is rarely required.

To stratify the risk of UGIB, scoring systems have been developed. Two commonly used systems are the Glasgow-Blatchford score and **AIMS65** score (online calculators are available for both systems). In 2011, Dr. John Saltzman published the AIMS65 scoring system. Calculating a score based on (A)lbumin, (I)NR, (M)ental status alteration, (S)ystolic blood pressure, and (65) age > 65 is simple and provides predictive mortality risk.

If significant GI bleeding is found, IV pantoprazole drip can be started. The octreotide bolus and drip should be started before endoscopy when variceal bleeding is suspected. With massive hematemesis, endotracheal tube intubation should be considered to protect the airway. Unless emergent endoscopy is planned, prokinetic drugs (erythromycin or metoclopramide) are not needed.

The differential diagnoses for upper GI bleeding include PUD, esophageal varices, esophagitis, Mallory Weiss tear, and vascular anomalies.

Disease	Bleeding Type	Association	Mortality
PUD	melena/hematemesis	NSAID use	5-10%
Esophageal varices	hematemesis	cirrhosis	10-15%
Esophagitis	hematemesis	heartburn	low
Mallory Weiss tear	hematemesis	retching	low
Vascular anomalies	melena/hematemesis	ESRD	low

Peptic ulcer is by far the most common cause of significant upper GI bleeding. Ulceration of the highly vascular stomach and duodenum can potentially lead to a life-threatening condition. NSAIDs, H. pylori infection, or stress ulceration are common causes. EGD can diagnose the issue, obtain tissue biopsy to evaluate for H.pylori, and perform immediate therapy (epinephrine injection, cautery of bleeding point, and endoscopic clips) to stop the bleeding.

The **risk of rebleeding** can be predicted based on the appearance of the ulcer. A clean based ulcer has low-risk, an adherent blood clot/pigmented material has a medium-risk, and an overtly bleeding or non-bleeding visible vessel have a high-risk for rebleeding.

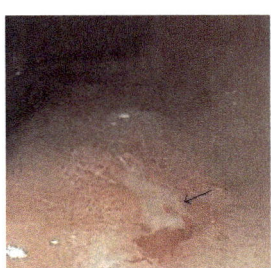
EGD: PUD with active bleeding

In cases of high-risk stigmata of rebleeding, PPI infusion should be continued for 72 hours, but an IV PPI drip is not usually necessary for low-risk ulcers. Oral PPI or once daily IV PPI is sufficient for ulcers with a low rebleeding risk.

Refractory bleeding from a duodenal ulcer can be treated with (IR) interventional radiology embolization of the gastroduodenal artery, which supplies blood flow to the duodenum. A reduction of blood flow after embolization can allow time for a duodenal ulcer to heal.

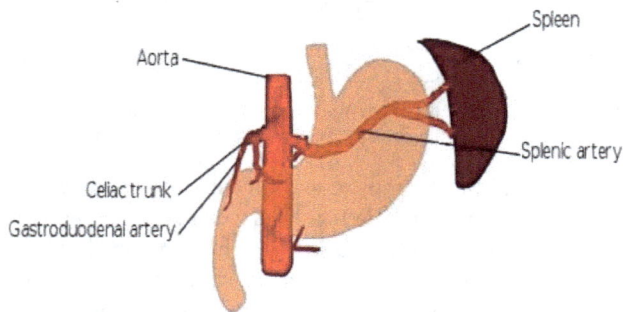

If medical, endoscopic, and radiologic methods fail, surgery with oversewing of the ulcer with an omental patch can be done.

Esophageal varices develop with increasing portal pressure. The most common reason is **liver cirrhosis.** With **portal hypertension**, pressure within the gastric veins increases, and blood flow distends the gastric and esophageal veins (esophageal varices).

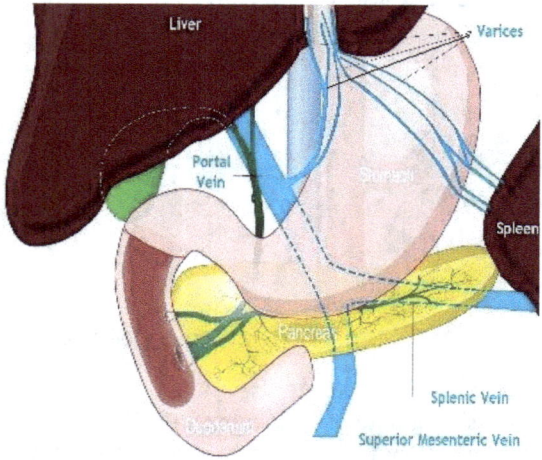

Variceal bleeding can lead to bacteremia. Therefore, start IV antibiotics to minimize the potential for spontaneous bacterial peritonitis. The risk of variceal rebleeding depends on the size of the varices and any high-risk stigmata. Upper endoscopy is needed to evaluate the varices.

Once varices are found, placement of rubber bands around the varices to ligate the vessels and stop bleeding is the preferred treatment. If esophageal varices rebleed, treatment with repeat endoscopy, placement of a fully covered esophageal stent (to compress the varices), placement of a Minnesota tube (to compress the varices, or interventional radiology placed TIPS (transjugular intrahepatic portosystemic shunt) are options.

Less commonly, variceal bleeding may occur from **gastric varices**. The underlying cause of gastric varices is different from esophageal varices. Splenic vein thrombosis related to acute pancreatitis is the most common cause of gastric varices. Gastric varices may also be related to a "spleno-renal vein shunt." With splenic vein thrombosis, the blood flow from the spleen cannot return to the liver by the splenic vein, and blood flow moves from the spleen into the smaller short gastric veins (resulting in gastric varices). The location of the splenic vein adjacent to the pancreas makes it susceptible to thrombosis from acute pancreatitis. Gastric varices can be large and have a potential for excessive bleeding.

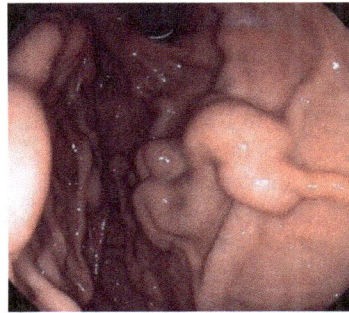 EGD: gastric varices

Gastric varices have been classified into four anatomic variants known as the Sarin classification: gastric esophageal varices 1, gastric esophageal varices 2, isolated gastric varices 1, and isolated gastric varices 2.

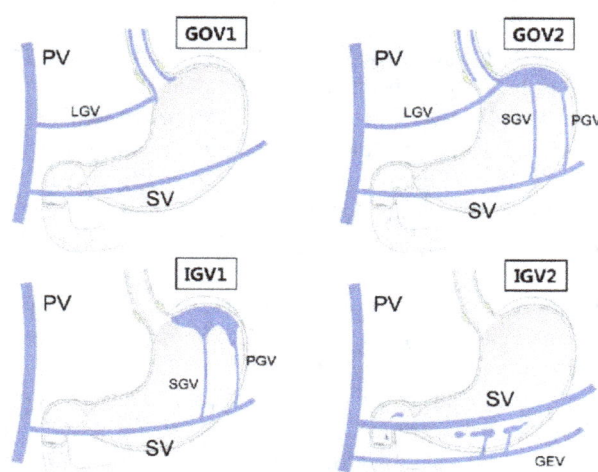

Endoscopic banding can be used for GOV1 and IGV2 varices. However, banding is likely ineffective for these varices. An exceedingly high mortality risk with GOV2 and IGV1 variceal bleeding requires more aggressive treatments. Treatment considerations include IR TIPS or an innovative IR procedure, coil-assisted retrograde transvenous obliteration (CARTO). Ultimately, splenectomy is the definitive treatment for GOV2 and IGV1 varices.

Esophagitis is usually related to GERD or regurgitation of gastric contents back into the esophagus. Esophageal bleeding presents with **hematemesis** (coffee ground appearance). Elderly bedridden patients are especially prone to esophagitis-induced bleeding; Endoscopy will confirm the diagnosis and deliver endoscopic therapy to stop any bleeding. Atypical-appearing esophagitis can be biopsied to evaluate for infection (CMV, HSV) or malignancy. PPI therapy is indicated for **reflux esophagitis**.

Mallory Weiss tear (MWT) is a mucosal tear at the gastroesophageal junction. It is commonly associated with significant vomiting/retching before the bleeding starts.

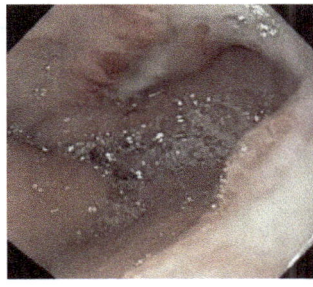
EGD: Mallory Weiss tear

MWT was first described by pathologists, Dr. Mallory and Dr. Weiss, in 1929 in a group of alcoholic patients with vomiting and hematemesis. The amount of bleeding is variable and can spontaneously heal. Endoscopic therapies are useful to reduce bleeding risk. The underlying cause of vomiting can be addressed, and PPI therapy is started to minimize acid reflux irritation of the tear.

Vascular lesions such as an arteriovenous malformation (AVM) or Dieulafoy vessel are common causes of upper GI bleeding. These conditions are associated with chronic renal disease, valvular heart disease, and/or hereditary hemorrhagic telangiectasia. At the capillary level, **AVMs** have an abnormally large connection between the arteriole and the venule. Increased pressure related to the larger connection can increase the tendency towards mucosal bleeding.

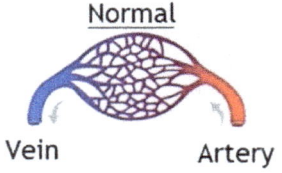
Normal
Vein   Artery

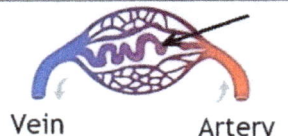
Arterial Venous Malformation
Vein   Artery

Dieulafoy vessel is an abnormally large caliber artery beneath the mucosa of the GI tract and is named for a French surgeon, Paul Georges Dieulafoy, who reported 10 cases of gastric bleeding in 1898. Dieulafoy arteries are believed to bleed once mucosal irritation or trauma causes a weakening of the overlying mucosa.[9] Most Dieulafoy bleeds are in the upper stomach near the gastroesophageal junction.

8. LOWER GI BLEED, Hematochezia

Take-Aways:

- *Diverticulosis is the most common cause of significant lower GI bleeding.*
- *Hemodynamics are critical. Do not rely on initial HGB/HCT to assess blood loss. IV fluid resuscitation is needed.*
- *Lower GI bleeding (red or maroon blood) frequently stops with supportive care.*
- *With significant bleeding, a CT angiogram can be done on presentation and may localize the bleeding source.*
- *Bowel prep prior to a colonoscopy is needed.*
- *Colon cancer must be excluded at some point with a colonoscopy.*

Hematochezia (red blood per rectum) is the hallmark of a lower GI bleed. Fortunately, lower GI bleeding usually is much less dangerous than upper GI bleeding. The bleeding source is usually from the colon, but occasionally small bowel bleeding results in LGIB. Increasing use of anticoagulants and antiplatelet agents increases the prevalence of bleeding. As such, the medication list is critical including aspirin, anticoagulants, and antiplatelet.

The color, rapidity of onset, and any associated pain are important descriptors. **Colonic bleeding** does not produce anal pain. Make sure to question females about vaginal bleeding as this could be mistaken for hematochezia. Previous colonoscopies or abdominal surgeries are important historical clues. The physical exam begins with an assessment of general appearance as a measure of toxicity. Resting vital signs are critical. A digital rectal exam is important to evaluate for hemorrhoids or perineal fistulas. Significant bleeding and signs of volume loss indicate the possibility of **a brisk upper GI bleed**. An EGD may need to occur with the colonoscopy to exclude an upper bleed.

Labs are important to assess coagulopathy and degree of anemia. **Imaging is not required for bleeding** unless abdominal pain is occurring as well. IV fluid resuscitation is critical. Generally, two large-bore peripheral IVs are suggested to increase fluids, blood transfusions, and medications as required. Acid suppression therapy **with PPI is unnecessary** for LGIB. If severely anemic, transfusion to a HGB of 8.0 mg/dl is suggested. **Coagulopathy should be corrected** by holding anticoagulants; and if active bleeding, transfuse fresh frozen plasma.

In cases of mild bleeding, begin a **bowel prep** to clear the blood from the colon. In general, an **unprepped emergent colonoscopy will not be helpful**. If significant acute bleeding is ongoing, CT angiogram with IV contrast can localize the source of bleeding, and **interventional radiology (IR) angiogram** with embolization of the blood vessel can stop bleeding. The American College of Gastroenterology 2023 clinical practice guideline recommends CT angiography as the initial diagnostic test for hemodynamically significant bleeding.[10]

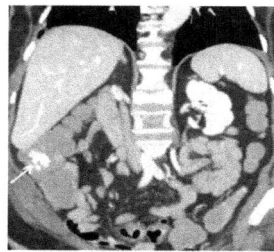

CTA: active GI bleeding

The **differential diagnosis** for lower GI bleeding includes diverticulosis, hemorrhoids, ischemic colitis, angiodysplasias, and infectious colitis. Colonoscopy is the test of choice; can determine the source, potentially stop the bleeding, and estimate prognosis.

Location	Bleeding Type	Association
Diverticulosis	red and/or clots	bleeding stops quickly
Hemorrhoids	red blood with bm	blood dripping into toilet
Ischemic colitis	red	abdominal pain;hx of cvd
Vascular lesions	red or maroon	elderly;renal disease
Infectious colitis	bloody diarrhea	diarrhea;hx of IBD

Diverticulosis is the most common cause of lower GI bleeding requiring hospitalization. Patients typically see a large amount of blood. Clinically, however, the amount of bleeding is not terribly severe. Diverticular pockets develop bulges outward, most commonly the sigmoid or descending colon, and the vascular supply to the diverticular mucosa is stretched down into the pockets. The edge and/or the base of the diverticula are prone to bleed (especially in patients on chronic aspirin therapy). Diverticular bleeding **will generally stop** with time, IV fluids, and holding of anticoagulants / antiplatelet agents. Patients should be made NPO and begin a bowel prep for colonoscopy in 1-2 days.

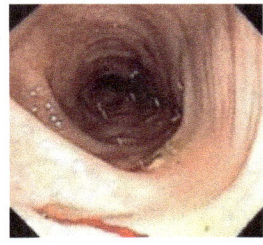 Colonoscopy: diverticular bleeding

Hemorrhoidal bleeding is usually painless red blood. Patients may notice a blood smear on a bowel movement or toilet tissue. When anal pain is present, suspect either an **external hemorrhoid** or an **anal fissure** (tear of the skin/mucosa). Patients may have other serious pathology in the colon even if hemorrhoidal bleeding occurs. If your patient has never had a colonoscopy, ensure a colonoscopy is done during hospitalization or in outpatient follow-up. **Colon cancer must be excluded** in cases of lower GI bleeding.

Ischemic colitis is common in elderly patients. Frequently, a previous history of cardiac or vascular disease will be present. In addition, anticoagulant or antiplatelet use can co-exist. Key features of ischemic colitis are **abdominal pain** and **bleeding**. Ischemic colitis is usually caused by microvascular changes but stenosis of the major branches of the superior mesenteric artery (SMA) or inferior mesenteric artery (IMA) can exist. Areas of ischemic colitis are the **"watershed areas"** of perfusion between the superior mesenteric, inferior mesenteric, and hemorrhoidal veins. The classic area for ischemic colitis bleeding is splenic flexure. Bleeding will usually resolve with IV hydration and time.

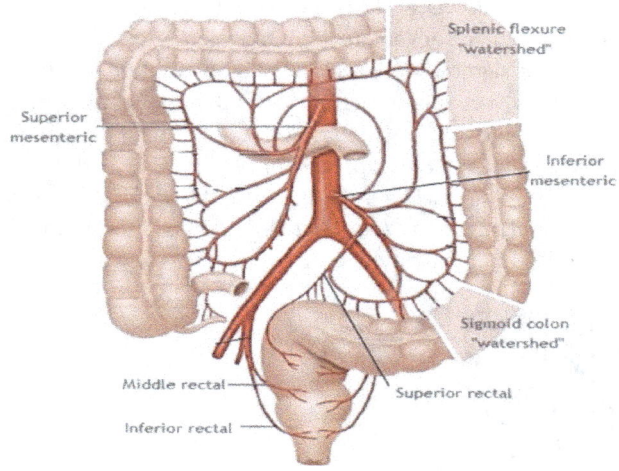

Vascular lesions can occur throughout the GI tract, as mentioned in the upper GI bleeding chapter, but they are also common in the small intestine or colon. The most common lesion is a mucosal arteriovenous malformation, an overlap of small arteries and veins with larger-than-normal vascular connections.

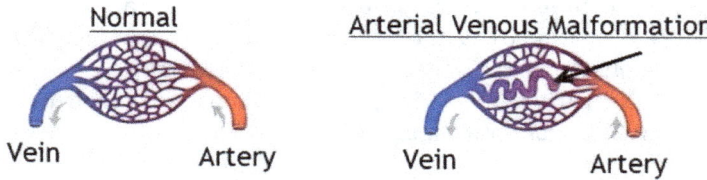

The small veins receive higher pressure related to the arterial connection. Increased pressure can lead to rupture and bleeding. **AVMs** are common in elderly and renal patients. Depending on the location, the bleeding can be red or maroon. If colonoscopy is unrevealing, a capsule endoscopy can be useful to evaluate the small bowel for acute bleeding.

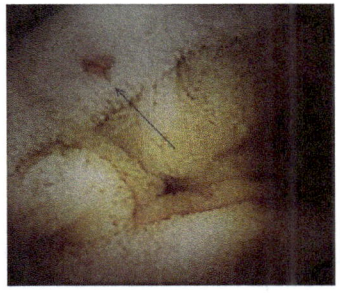 Capsule endoscopy: ileal AVM

Colitis is the inflammation of the colon, usually from an acute infection. Dysentery is the common term for a bacterial colonic infection with bloody diarrhea. Inflammatory bowel disease, either ulcerative colitis or Crohn's disease, is another cause of lower GI bleeding. Radiation colitis or medication-induced colitis are rare causes of bleeding.

9. Jaundice / Increased Liver Enzymes

Take-Aways:

- *Jaundice can be classified as conjugated or unconjugated.*
- *The pattern and severity of AST/ALT elevation is important. ALT is primarily produced in the liver.*
- *Pt/INR is a good measure of liver synthetic function. An increasing INR is worrisome for liver failure.*
- *Painless jaundice is worrisome for pancreatic or biliary malignancy. Exclude pancreatic cancer with painless jaundice.*

Jaundice is yellow discoloration of the skin that occurs when the bilirubin elevates >3.0 mg/dl. Liver enzyme elevations can be asymptomatic or have corresponding symptoms of the underlying disease. Patients with viral syndrome may complain of fatigue, malaise, or myalgias. Rarely vomiting, itching, or upper abdominal pain can occur related to swelling of the liver and stretching of the liver capsule. Past medical and social history are important. Prescription, over the counter, and herbal supplements are important as drug-induced liver disease **(DILI)** is quite common. Obesity and other features of the metabolic syndrome can lead to gallbladder and nonalcoholic fatty liver disease **(NAFLD)**. Pregnancy or recent pregnancy is associated with gallstones and other pregnancy-specific liver diseases as well.

Patient behaviors like EtOH and illicit drug use can be contributing factors. Tattoos, body piercings, and sexual exposure are risk factors for viral liver disease. Travel, work, and environmental exposure are important if a water or food-borne illness is possible. Finally, a **family history** of liver disease, celiac disease, or inflammatory bowel disease could point to a familial disorder.

Begin your examination with observation. Look for signs of liver disease, such as jaundice, icterus, xanthelasma, palmar erythema, spider angiomata, gynecomastia, ascites, liver enlargement, enlargement of the spleen, testicular atrophy, asterixis, or confusion.

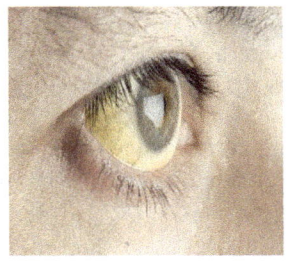
Icterus

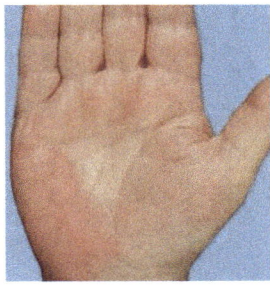
Palmar erythema

AST and ALT are **hepatocellular indicators** and suggest irritation or damage to hepatocytes. AST is produced from the liver, muscle, and the kidney. ALT is more specific to the liver. Chronic EtOH use elevates the AST more than ALT. Frequently, **AST/ALT ratio** will be > 2. Bilirubin and alkaline phosphatase are primarily measures of liver **conjugation** and **excretion of bilirubin**. Albumin and total protein are measures of liver **synthetic function**.

In addition, **Pt/INR** is the best clinical measure of changing liver **synthetic function**. Since the INR is an indirect measure of the vitamin K-dependent factors of coagulation (including factor VII with a short half-life of 3-6 hours), measuring the INR daily or perhaps twice daily can be considered to monitor patients with suspected acute liver failure.

The list of liver serologic tests is extensive, but for inpatient evaluation, minimum testing includes **acute hepatitis panel, EtOH level, ANA, acetaminophen level, urine drug screen, and iron/TIBC**. In certain cases, TSH, monospot, EBV, CMV, Hep E antigen, or HSV titers could be useful.

Ultrasound is the test of choice to evaluate the liver and gallbladder. Frequently, hepatic Doppler is added to evaluate the patency of the hepatic vessels and the direction of flow. Doppler is useful if portal vein thrombosis, hepatic vein thrombosis (Budd-Chiari Syndrome), or portal hypertension is suspected. An MRCP, endoscopic ultrasound, or ERCP can be performed in cases of suspected biliary tract obstruction. Tissue diagnosis with a **liver biopsy is rarely needed** for the inpatient workup.

The most efficient method to investigate jaundice is to divide the elevation into either **conjugated (direct)** or **unconjugated (indirect)** hyperbilirubinemia. The liver conjugates bilirubin by combining it with glucuronic acid to make it water-soluble. The water-soluble bilirubin can then be excreted from the liver into the bile ducts. A portion of bilirubin covalently binds to albumin, known as "delta bilirubin." Delta bilirubin will persist until the bound albumin is cleared. Jaundice may persist for a few days after other LFTs improve.

Conjugated bilirubin is usually due to extrahepatic biliary obstruction from stone disease or malignancy but can be related to intrahepatic cholestasis related to acute viral hepatitis, primary biliary cirrhosis, primary sclerosing cholangitis, long-term TPN, drugs like oral contraceptives, amoxicillin/clavulanate, and clopidogrel.

Unconjugated bilirubin is usually related to bilirubin overproduction/release (hemolysis) or ineffective erythropoiesis (thalassemia, lead toxicity). **LDH** and **haptoglobin** are useful for evaluating hemolysis. Impaired bilirubin uptake can be caused by congestive heart failure or drugs (rifampin, aspirin, NSAIDs). Impaired conjugation of bilirubin can be an underlying inherited deficiency like **Gilbert's syndrome** (3-5% of the population, the majority are men), which is a benign condition causing jaundice with stress, illness, or dehydration.

Disease	LFT Pattern	Association
Biliary obstruction	bilirubin;alk phos	CBD stone;pancreas mass
Acute viral hepatitis	AST;ALT	viral illness with fatigue
Drug induced	mixed	acetaminophen
EtOH liver disease	AST ratio to alt >2:1	increased GGT
Shock liver	↑ ↑ ↑ AST&ALT	sepsis;hypotension

Biliary tract obstruction is usually related to the passage of biliary stones into the common bile duct. Head of pancreas and biliary malignancies can also lead to this pattern of elevated bilirubin with an increase in alkaline phosphatase. Biliary stones usually involve RUQ pain. In cases of **painless jaundice, malignancy** must be excluded. When there is acute pancreatitis, jaundice or LFT abnormalities can occur from CBD compression.

Gallstones are more common in fertile women under age forty related to hormones. The **"3F"** phrase of female, fertile, and under forty is an easy memory aid. In addition, Native Americans and Hispanic persons have an increased risk of gallstones. In cases of jaundice or suspected biliary obstruction, ultrasound frequently reveals clues such as gallstones, a dilated common bile duct, or rarely even a bile duct stone. However, bile duct stones are difficult to visualize on routine ultrasound. Follow-up endoscopic testing should be considered with either **EUS** or **ERCP**.

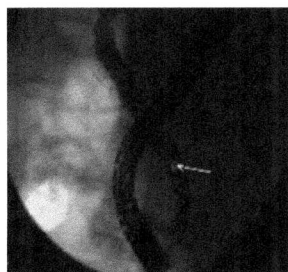
ERCP: bile duct stone

In general, if bilirubin or alkaline phosphatase is elevated and CBD is dilated, proceed to ERCP. If endoscopy is not chosen, MRCP can help exclude CBD abnormalities. HIDA scan evaluates the patency of the cystic and common bile ducts. HIDA can be useful when other tests are inconclusive.

Jean-Martin Charcot (1825-1893) reported a triad of conditions (fever, RUQ pain, and jaundice) associated with "intermittent biliary fever" in 1877. **Charcot's triad** is still a useful eponym, but cholangitis is our modern terminology for infection within the bile duct. Cholangitis warrants an **ERCP within 48-72 hours of presentation** to remove obstruction and/or drain infection from the bile duct. Delayed ERCP (>72 hours) is associated with more complications, longer hospital stays, and higher mortality.[11] Another study has shown that ERCP performed within 24 hours of presentation for acute cholangitis has a lower 30-day mortality rate.[12] A general recommendation is that ERCP should be performed within 48 hours for cholangitis.

Acute viral hepatitis usually presents with a prodromal illness: fatigue, fever, anorexia, and malaise. Exposure to contaminated food or water sources can lead to acute hepatitis A or E. Blood exposure (IVDA is a common example) or sexual exposure can lead to acute hepatitis B or C. Mononucleosis, CMV, and HSV acute hepatitis are considerations as well. The AST and ALT can be dramatically elevated (5 -10x). Psychosocial history will give you powerful clues. Treatment is supportive, and the PT/INR is monitored to look for signs of decompensation of liver function.

Drug-induced liver injury is common. The classic description is from acetaminophen toxicity. However, other common medications like amiodarone, HMG CoA inhibitors, phenytoin, carbamazepine, oral contraceptives, clopidogrel, nitrofurantoin, and fluconazole can lead to liver injury. **Over the counter** drugs like ephedra, senna, and NSAIDs are also known causes. Illicit drugs like ecstasy and cocaine can elevate the LFTs. Once other causes have been excluded, treatment is withholding any potential drugs that may have caused the liver disease.

EtOH liver disease is usually obvious in an acutely intoxicated patient. However, highly functioning patients can conceal EtOH abuse, and women are particularly susceptible to EtOH-related liver injury. Elevation of AST out of proportion to ALT **(usually >2:1 ratio)** and the elevation of GGT are clues. EtOH level should be obtained on admission. The bilirubin and INR can be increased in severe EtOH hepatitis. Treatment is supportive with observation for withdrawal and encouragement of alcoholic anonymous/rehab programs.

In cases of severe EtOH hepatitis, steroids can be helpful. The **discriminant function (Maddrey score)** can be used to estimate the severity of liver damage. Discriminant function calculation is prothrombin time minus the control prothrombin time multiplied by the 4.6 plus the total bilirubin(PT-control PT) x 4.6 + total bili). If the discriminant function is **>32, steroids** should be considered.

Ischemic hepatitis (shock liver) is a consideration when dramatic elevations of the AST and ALT occur. Cases of trauma, sepsis, and severe congestive heart failure can result in under-perfusion of the liver. Monitoring for signs of acute liver failure and supportive care are standard treatments, and LFT will generally improve with improvement of the underlying condition.

10. Ascites/Cirrhosis

Take-Aways:

- *Ascites is a sign of decompensated liver disease.*
- *Serum to ascites albumin gradient can differentiate etiologies. Rarely, ascites may have non-hepatic causes.*
- *MELD and Child's score provide prognostic information.*
- *Complications of cirrhosis (GI bleeding, hepatic encephalopathy, and ascites) are frequent causes of hospitalization.*

Ascites is fluid accumulation within the peritoneum. The most common cause is liver cirrhosis. With scarring (cirrhosis), blood flow through the liver is altered, and portal vein pressure increases. Portal hypertension, vasodilation of the gut circulation, and increased hydrostatic pressure can lead to leakage (weeping) of ascites into the peritoneum.

EtOH abuse is the classic cause of cirrhosis. However, other etiologies such as nonalcoholic fatty liver disease (NAFLD), hepatitis B and C, and autoimmune hepatitis exist. Ascites, hepatic encephalopathy, variceal bleeding, and renal failure are the common complications of liver disease requiring hospitalization. **Ascites is a poor prognostic sign**. In general, once ascites develops, a high mortality within 2 years is expected. Abdominal swelling, lower extremity edema, and weight gain are also common symptoms. Occasionally, shortness of breath can occur.

Past **medical history** and social history provide important context. Medications, including prescription, over the counter, or herbal supplements, are valuable to understanding the overall health of your patient. **Obesity** and features of metabolic **syndrome** are common. Patient behaviors like EtOH use and illicit drug use may be contributing factors. Tattoos, body piercings, and sexual exposure are important historical clues. Finally, any family history of liver disease, celiac disease, or inflammatory bowel disease should be noted.

Jaundice, icterus, xanthelasma, palmar erythema, spider angiomata, gynecomastia, ascites, liver enlargement, enlargement of the spleen, testicular atrophy, asterixis, and/or confusion may be exam findings with cirrhosis.

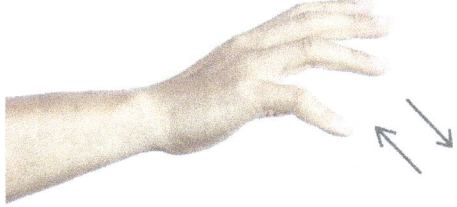

Asterixis

With ascites, the flanks may bulge. Ascitic fluid is dull to percussion and may shift with patient movement. Initial labs include BMP, CBC, LFT, and Pt/INR.

Ultrasound is the test of choice for evaluating the liver and ascites. Hepatic Doppler can be added to assess the patency of hepatic vessels and the direction of blood flow. If a liver mass is suspected, CT with IV contrast (liver mass protocol) will be helpful. A CT scan of the abdomen can be considered. A right pleural effusion, hepatic hydrothorax, can develop from ascites moving from the abdomen into the right pleural space via small defects of the diaphragm.

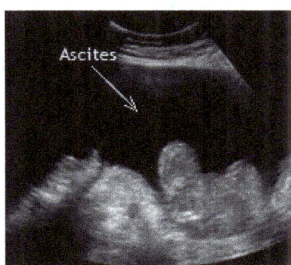

Ultrasound: ascites

New or symptomatic ascites warrants a **paracentesis** for fluid analysis and to exclude infection. The fluid is usually light yellow in color. If white in color, one should suspect chylous ascites (check the triglyceride level in the fluid). Laboratory testing of ascitic fluid can narrow the causes of ascites. The key calculation is the **serum to ascites albumin gradient** (SAAG). Since the ascites fluid has a low albumin content, the SAAG is particularly useful. Serum albumin minus the ascites albumin is ≥1.1 in cases of liver-related ascites. Other diagnostic tests include culture and cell count, total protein, and cytology. In rare cases, the fluid can be sent for amylase, LDH, triglyceride, and AFB stain/culture.

In practice, routinely send fluid to your lab for **cell count with differential, culture, albumin, and total protein**. Additional fluid can be sent to the lab and held for 24-28 hours. If unexpected initial results develop, other tests can be obtained without the need for a repeat paracentesis.

Etiology	SAAG	Total Protein	Color	Association
Cirrhosis	≥1.1	<2.5	yellow	SBP
Acute Hepatitis	≥1.1	<2.5	yellow	EtOH use
CHF	≥1.1	>2.5	yellow	LE edema
Malignancy	<1.1	>2.5	cloudy	ovarian cancer
Tuberculosis	<1.1	>2.5	cloudy	prior TB infection

Ascites severity can be divided into three segments. **Grade 1** ascites is mild and only found on imaging, **Grade 2** ascites is moderate and present on physical exam, and **Grade 3** is severe with large ascites with a distended abdomen. Complications of ascites include the development of infection (spontaneous bacterial peritonitis), a right pleural effusion (hepatic hydrothorax), and rarely renal failure (hepatorenal syndrome).

Cirrhotic ascites is the most common (>75% of cases). SAAG will be high, the total protein level will be low, and the fluid will usually be clear to yellow. Spontaneous bacterial peritonitis **(SBP)** must be excluded; the most reliable diagnostic measure is the polymorphonuclear cells (PMN) in the fluid.

If > 250 PMN are present, SBP should be treated. In addition, ascitic fluid can be sent to microbiology (in blood culture bottles) for culture. However, cultures are frequently negative.

Treatment guidelines for cirrhotic ascites without infection are a 2-gram sodium-restricted diet and consideration of diuretic therapy (spironolactone/furosemide). Other complications of cirrhosis include portal HTN, bleeding from esophageal varices or portal HTN gastropathy, confusion from hepatic encephalopathy, hepatorenal syndrome, and hepatocellular carcinoma.

A potentially severe complication from acute or chronic liver disease is **severe renal dysfunction**. With acute liver dysfunction, decreased blood flow to the kidneys can result in severe acute kidney injury. Volume replacement with IV fluids and albumin are frequently used as a "colloid" to expand intravascular volume. Cirrhosis can also cause low systemic blood pressure with reduced renal perfusion. Midodrine is frequently used to increase systemic blood pressure as an adjunct to increasing renal perfusion. With volume expansion and normalization of systemic blood pressure, **increased renal perfusion** can occur and reverse acute kidney injury.

Hepatorenal syndrome (HRS) may be present if persistent renal failure exists after volume expansion. HRS is a dreaded condition with an exceedingly high mortality. Two subtypes of hepatorenal syndrome exist. **Type 1 HRS** has a quick onset of increasing creatinine over 10-14 days. Urine output also drops significantly. **Type 2 HRS** is a slower increase of creatinine and frequently results in an increase in ascites and progressive overall fluid retention.

Treatment for HRS is focused on improving intravascular blood flow to the kidneys. Octreotide and midodrine are medical options. If medical treatment fails, IR TIPS placement is a good treatment option. However, HRS is frequently **progressive**. Dialysis can be started IF a liver transplant is a possibility. Consultation with a liver transplant team should be done prior to starting dialysis. If your patient is not a transplant candidate, dialysis should not be considered.

Estimating the severity of liver disease/cirrhosis is challenging. However, two scoring systems have been shown to have clinical utility: **MELD** and **Child's-Pugh Score**: MELD (Model of End Stage Liver Disease) was originally developed at Mayo Clinic and has been shown to be predictive of a 3-month survival. MELD is a calculation based on the patient's bilirubin, creatinine, and INR. The addition of serum sodium is labeled as **MELD-Na**. Online calculators or apps are available to perform the MELD calculation.

MELD	3-month Mortality
<9	2%
10-19	6%
20-29	20%
30-39	52%
>40	71%

Child's-Pugh scoring system uses five clinical measures of liver disease. For each measure, a score of 1-3 is given. The total score provides prognostic information.[13]

Child-Pugh score variables	1 Point	2 Points	3 Points
Total bilirubin	<2	2-3	>3
Albumin	>3.5	3.5-2.8	<2.8
INR	<1.7	1.7-2.3	>2.3
Ascites	None	Mild	Moderate
Hepatic Encephalopathy	None	I-II	III-IV

Total Child's Score	Grade	1yr mortality	2yr mortality
5–6	A	100%	85%
7–9	B	81%	57%
10–15	C	45%	35%

11. Acute Liver Failure

Take-Aways:

- *Liver injury with coagulopathy and a mental status change defines acute liver failure.*
- *Acetaminophen overdose is a classic cause of acute liver failure. EtOH increases the toxic effect of acetaminophen.*
- *Viral hepatitis and severe alcoholic hepatitis are also potential causes. Autoimmune hepatitis is a rare cause of acute liver failure.*
- *Acute liver failure has a high morbidity and mortality.*

Acute liver failure is associated with **coagulopathy** (INR > 1.5) and **confusion.** Intense inflammation and/or hepatic necrosis result in reduced synthesis of clotting factors and coagulopathy related to the short half-life of vitamin K-dependent clotting factors (Factor VII $t_{1/2}$ = 6 hours). **Mental status changes** (hepatic encephalopathy) develop, and cerebral edema can also occur. Presenting complaints can be **vague symptoms** like fatigue, confusion, nausea, or lack of appetite. Overt signs of liver disease like ascites, icterus, or jaundice may not be present. Past medical and social history are important clues for potential causes.

Medications including prescription, over the counter, or herbal supplements are important as drug-induced liver disease (DILI) is quite common. **Acetaminophen** intake must be questioned. Patient behaviors like smoking, smokeless tobacco use, EtOH, and illicit drug use can be contributing factors. Tattoos, body piercings, and sexual exposure are important historical clues. Specific causes of acute liver failure are related to pregnancy or recent pregnancy. Travel, work, and environmental exposure may explain a recent infectious hepatitis. Jaundice, icterus, ascites, hepatomegaly, and/or confusion could be present. The baseline and evolving neurologic exam should be followed.

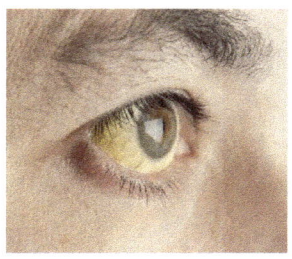
Icterus

Hepatic encephalopathy is a sign of liver deterioration which can manifest with signs ranging from insomnia and irritability to confusion and coma.

Hepatic encephalopathy grading	
Grade I	mild psychomotor slowing, mood changes insomnia
Grade II	mild confusion, asterixis
Grade III	marked confusion, lethargy, will wake to verbal stimuli
Grade IV	coma, will not wake even to painful stimuli

LFTs, CBC, PT/INR, BMP, acute hepatitis panel, acetaminophen level, urine drug screen, EtOH level, ANA, and urine pregnancy testing are indicated for initial evaluation. Periodic measurement of Pt/INR is needed to monitor liver synthetic function.

Ultrasound is the test of choice for liver and potential ascites. Frequently, **hepatic doppler** is used to evaluate the patency of the hepatic vessels and direction of flow. As part of acute liver failure evaluation, the potential for liver transplant candidacy must be addressed as well. Consultation with the nearest liver transplant center is wise. Avoid sedatives, if possible since mental status changes need to be monitored. Cerebral edema may develop with worsening encephalopathy. Signs/symptoms of cerebral edema include increased systemic blood pressure, bradycardia, and respiratory depression. ICU monitoring and/or transfer to a liver transplant center are considerations.

In addition to clinical assessment, objective data can guide when to consider liver transplantation. Guidelines from the United Kingdom (Kings College) list transplant consideration guidelines for acetaminophen and other causes of acute liver failure. Again, consultation with the nearest liver transplant program is suggested.

Kings College Transplantation Guidelines for Acute Liver Failure:	
Acetaminophen	Arterial ph< 7.30 *or* PT > 100 + creatinine >3.4 mg/dl + grade III/IV encephalopathy
Not Acetaminophen	PT >100 *or* Any three of the following: Drug induced liver failure, Jaundice to coma < 7 days, PT > 50, Bilirubin > 17.5, Age <10 or >40 yr

Acetaminophen is the most common cause of acute liver failure and has a dose-dependent toxicity. Overdose can be accidental or intentional. Toxicity usually requires greater than 5000 mg of a single dose or repeated days of more than 4000 mg/day. **Underlying alcoholic liver disease** predisposes to acetaminophen toxicity due to the upregulation of cytochrome P450 (CYP 2E1), which promotes an increase in acetaminophen toxic metabolites. An antidote, n-acetylcysteine **(NAC)** is available. N-acetylcysteine should be started within 24 hours of ingestion. Get an acetaminophen level upon presentation to determine if a toxic amount of acetaminophen has been ingested.[14] Closely monitor mentation, daily LFTs, INR, and electrolytes. Recovery from acetaminophen toxicity is associated with electrolyte abnormalities, especially **magnesium and phosphorus**.

Etiology	AST:ALT	Association	Treatment
Acetaminophen	>500	EtOH use	N-acetylcysteine
Acute Viral Hepatitis	>500	IVDA	Supportive
Ischemic Hepatitis	>500	Sepsis trauma	Treat cause
EtOH Liver Disease	<500	AST/ALT >2	Steroids
Drug Induced	<500	Mixed LFTs elevation	Remove drug

Acute viral hepatitis is related to hepatitis A, B, C, D, E, HSV, CMV. Risk factors for hepatitis B, C, and D include parenteral transmission with **blood or sexual contact**. Hepatitis A and E are spread by oral transmission with food or water. Infection with acute hepatitis D in a patient with chronic hepatitis B; or acute hepatitis E in pregnancy carries a substantial mortality. All cases of moderate or severe elevations of the AST/ALT should have an acute hepatitis panel. **Hepatitis C antibodies may take 6-12 weeks to become positive.** Therefore, a patient with acute liver failure and a positive hepatitis C antibody likely has chronic hepatitis C and another cause of acute liver failure. Physical exam frequently reveals icterus and jaundice. Treatment is supportive. Acute hepatitis B can be treated with direct acting nucleoside analogs. Hepatitis A does not cause chronic liver disease.

Ischemic hepatitis or "shock liver" is a common cause of acute liver failure in conditions such as sepsis, trauma, acute cardiac events, or massive bleeding. The underlying injury is from decreased blood flow and decreased oxygen delivery to the liver; oxygen delivery to the liver is highly dependent upon cardiac function.

Right heart failure is a frequent cause or contributor to ischemic hepatitis.[15] The liver receives blood flow by the portal vein (approximately 2/3 flow) and by the hepatic artery (approximately 1/3). The LFT can be dramatically increased (AST/ALT > 1000 mg/dl) with ischemic hepatitis.

EtOH liver disease can result in liver failure with severe acute EtOH hepatitis. Acute liver damage from EtOH is accompanied by abdominal pain, jaundice, nausea, and anorexia. As with all cases of liver failure, monitor for confusion and coagulopathy. EtOH liver disease patients routinely receive replacement **of thiamine, folate, magnesium, and multivitamins**. Mild cases of EtOH hepatitis will resolve with time and avoidance of EtOH.

For moderate or severe cases of EtOH liver disease, medications are advised. Severity of liver injury in acute EtOH hepatitis can be determined with the **discriminant function (Maddrey Score)**. Calculation is easy and predictive of 30-day mortality.

Use the following formula: (**Patient PT– Lab Control PT) x 4.6 + Total bilirubin**. When the discriminant function is greater **than 32, methylprednisolone 40 mg daily for one month** has been shown to reduce 30-day mortality. The steroids are tapered over two weeks afterward. Pentoxifylline was used in the past. However, pentoxifylline has been proven to be ineffective and is no longer used.

Drug induced liver injury (DILI). Drug reactions can be dose-dependent or idiosyncratic (not dose-dependent). In addition, a patient can be taking medication for months without toxicity before the drug reaction occurs. The list of potential medications implicated in DILI is extensive and includes NSAIDs, amiodarone, amoxicillin/clavulanate, phenytoin, and valproic acid. Over the counter and/or herbal products such as Herbalife, Hydroxycut, and ephedra have also been reported as causes of DILI. The treatment is supportive care and removal of the drug.

12. Pancreatitis / Increased Lipase

Take-Aways:

- *Lipase is more specific to the pancreas than amylase.*
- *Pancreatitis is commonly caused by passage of gallstones / biliary sludge or EtOH abuse.*
- *Lipase may not be increased with chronic pancreatitis.*
- *Rarely, severe peptic ulcer disease can mimic acute pancreatitis.*
- *Pancreatic tumors can mimic symptoms of pancreatitis.*

Lipase is a digestive enzyme that aids in the digestion of fat. Most lipase is produced from the pancreas, but lesser amounts are produced in the stomach and intestine. When compared to amylase, **lipase has a longer half-life and is more specific to the pancreas.** An asymptomatic increased lipase may not indicate pancreatitis.

Acute pancreatitis is a painful condition in which premature activation of trypsinogen and release of inflammatory cytokines result. As a result, increased pancreatic enzymes are formed leading to some autodigestion of the pancreas. Acute pancreatitis causes diffuse edema, hemorrhage, or even significant destruction of the pancreas (**necrotizing pancreatitis**). Acute pancreatitis causes over 250,000 hospital admissions each year in the US.[16] Symptoms of **pancreatitis** include abdominal pain, nausea, and/or vomiting. The duration of upper abdominal symptoms is helpful when considering pancreatitis.

Acute pancreatitis is **quite painful**. Pain usually originates in the epigastrium and frequently radiates to the back. Previous surgical history (cholecystectomy) and social history(EtOH and tobacco) are especially important. **Smoking is an underrecognized risk factor**. Synergistic effects of alcohol and smoking as a cause of acute pancreatitis do exist.[17] Rarely, pancreatitis can be hereditary.

On exam, the vital signs can point to toxicity. **Significant intravascular volume depletion** can occur. Resting tachycardia signals the need for volume replacement with **IV fluids** (lactate ringers is preferred over normal saline). A patient who is restless and uncomfortable is suggestive of pancreatitis. In addition, patients may find relief by leaning forward in the seated position. If bluish discoloration in the flanks (Gray Turner sign) or periumbilical area (Cullen sign) is present, the patient may have hemorrhagic pancreatitis.

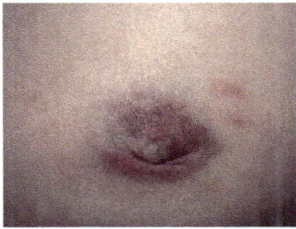 Cullen's sign

Labs include a complete blood count, basic metabolic panel, liver function, and lipase. In addition, serum triglyceride level is useful. A lipase elevation of <u>**at least 3 times the normal range**</u> with abdominal pain consistent with pancreatitis is needed to diagnose acute pancreatitis.[18] Alternatively, **radiologic findings of pancreatitis** coupled with abdominal pain is also diagnostic of acute pancreatitis.

Common imaging includes abdominal ultrasound and CT. Ultrasound is the test of choice for suspected gallstones. The presence of stones, biliary sludge, or gallbladder wall inflammation/pericholecystic fluid suggests acute cholecystitis.

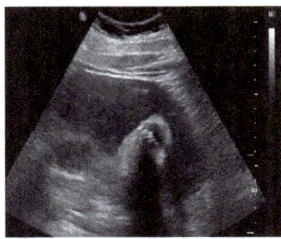 Ultrasound: stone with shadow

Computed tomography is the most used imaging technique. MRI can be used for the pancreas and is especially useful for evaluating the common bile duct and pancreatic duct (MRCP protocol).

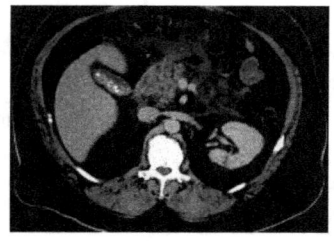
CT: pancreatitis

Disease	Pain Location	Pain Severity	Association
Acute Pancreatitis	epigastric back	high	back pain
Chronic Pancreatitis	epigastric	variable	diarrhea
Pancreatic Tumor	epigastric back	variable	wt loss
Peptic Ulcer Disease	RUQ epigastric	variable	NSAIDs

Common **causes of acute pancreatitis** are gallstones/gallbladder sludge, EtOH, hypertriglyceridemia, hypercalcemia, and ERCP. The passage of gallstones or biliary sludge through the common bile duct into the duodenum can cause mechanical pressure on the pancreatic duct resulting in acute pancreatitis. EtOH use can cause chronic inflammation of the pancreas. **Hypertriglyceridemia** pancreatitis occurs via the breakdown of fat in the pancreas, causing inflammation from free fatty acids. Usually, the serum triglyceride levels are > 1000mg/dl. Elevated levels of calcium are theorized to cause premature activation of trypsinogen in the pancreas resulting in auto-digestion.[19]

Acute pancreatitis can be mild with a short hospital stay or severe with ICU care and life-threatening complications. Systemic complications like acute kidney injury and respiratory distress can occur early. Late complications, including pancreatic fluid collections(walled-off necrosis and pseudocyst), are possible.

Several scoring systems can estimate the prognosis of acute pancreatitis. The most used are the Ranson criteria and the modified Balthazar CT severity index.

The original **Ranson criteria** is a predictive system developed by Dr. John Ranson at New York University Medical Center in 1974. The system requires measuring 5 criteria on admission and evaluating other signs 48 hours after admission. The total score is tabulated after 48 hours.

Ranson Criteria		
Admission	48 hrs after admission	Total score
age> 55	calcium <8.0	0-2 : 2% mortality
glucose>200	HCT drop <10%	3-4 : 15% mortality
AST > 250	PaO2 < 60	5-6 : 40% mortality
LDH > 350	BUN increase > 5 fluid Sequestration > 6L	7-8 : 100% mortality

CT Severity Index (CTSI) is a radiologic scoring system for assessing the severity of acute pancreatitis. The index was developed by Dr. Emil Balthazar in 1994 to measure the level of pancreatic inflammation and was later modified to include the degree of pancreatic necrosis.[21]

Grade of Pancreatitis	Score	Necrosis	Score
normal	0	None	0
enlarged pancreas	1	<30%	2
inflamed peripancreatic fat	2	>30-50%	4
single fluid collection	3	>50%	6
more than one fluid collection	4		

Interpretation (Grade of Pancreatitis Score + Necrosis Score)

0-3: mild pancreatitis

4-6: moderate pancreatitis

7-10: severe pancreatitis

Acute pancreatitis is treated with **IV fluids** and pain and nausea medications. In contrast to prior recommendations, early feeding with at least liquids in the first 24 hours is suggested. Antibiotics are unnecessary for mild pancreatitis. Severe pancreatitis warrants ICU monitoring, aggressive IV fluids, and patient-controlled pain medication. Antibiotic use for severe pancreatitis is controversial. Feeding by mouth or nasoenteral tube is needed if your patient cannot take food by mouth. **IV nutrition (TPN) should rarely be used.** The lipase level will fluctuate during pancreatitis and does not correlate with disease severity. **Daily monitoring of the lipase is not recommended.**

Chronic Pancreatitis involves chronic inflammation and fibrosis of the pancreatic tissue and calcifications can occur. Patients become symptomatic with diarrhea when <20% of pancreatic exocrine function remains. Common causes are EtOH abuse, idiopathic, autoimmune, hereditary, obstructed pancreatic duct, and prior acute pancreatitis.

Symptoms of **chronic dull pain**, diarrhea, steatorrhea, and weight loss can occur. Nausea and anorexia are possible. **Exam is often unimpressive** to the degree of pain the patient reports.[22,23] Rarely, icterus and jaundice occur. Labs are generally unrevealing with a mild increase in WBC and occasional increase in LFTs, and the lipase can be normal or only minimally elevated. X-rays can show calcifications of the pancreas.

CT or MR imaging may reveal a dilated pancreatic duct.[24] ERCP or endoscopic ultrasound frequently have distinct findings but are not needed for hospital care. Stool elastase is useful for evaluating decreased pancreatic exocrine function. Treatment is primarily directed toward symptom control of pain, nausea, and dehydration. Pancreatic enzyme replacement reduces the degree of diarrhea and maldigestion. Endoscopic therapy with PD stone removal, drainage of pancreatic fluid collections, and/or celiac plexus block may be indicated in certain situations.

Tumors of the pancreas can be malignant or benign. The most common malignant tumor is adenocarcinoma. **With painless jaundice pancreatic cancer must be excluded.** With pancreatic ductal involvement, abdominal pain, and increased lipase can occur. Symptomatic lesions are usually 2-3 cm in size, located in the head of the pancreas (large enough to compress something), and frequently metastatic to local or regional nodes. Tumors in the tail of pancreas may get much larger before causing symptoms (5-6 cm).

When presenting with **back pain, metastatic extension to the retroperitoneum** is usually present. Major risk factors include a family history of pancreatic cancer and smoking. After initial diagnosis, definitive staging is done as an outpatient. After staging, consultation with medical and surgical oncologists is needed to consider surgical resection for cure, chemotherapy, or endoscopic rx for palliation.

Benign lesions like **pancreatic cysts** are possible. Benign lesions are usually in the elderly and are often found incidentally on CT imaging. When a lesion is found, differentiating between a malignancy and a benign is the primary objective. **CA 19-9** lab is a tumor marker associated with pancreaticobiliary cancers, but CA 19-9 is not diagnostic of cancer. Imaging with a CT scan, MRI, Endoscopic ultrasound, and/or ERCP can be done.

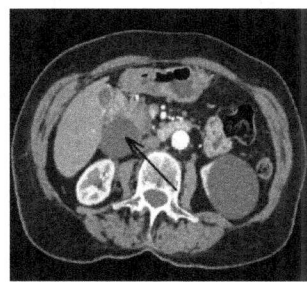 CT: benign pancreatic cyst

Gastric or duodenal ulcers can cause pain like pancreatitis and may mildly increase the lipase. Rarely, ulcers will erode and penetrate the pancreas itself. The most common etiologies for gastric and duodenal ulcers are H. pylori and NSAID use. With suspected PUD, an EGD can confirm or rule out ulcers.

13. Inflammatory Bowel Disease: Crohn's / Ulcerative Colitis

Take-Aways:

- *IBD is an abnormally aggressive immune response to normal intestinal contents.*
- *IBD has two major phenotypes, Crohn's and ulcerative colitis.*
- *Crohn's involvement has skip area and is commonly located in the ileum or colon.*
- *Ulcerative colitis starts in the rectum and can extend upward continuously to the cecum, and ulcerative colitis is only located in the colon.*
- *IBD is a lifelong condition characterized by intermittent flares. Despite improved medical treatments, IBD patients may need surgery at some point in their life.*

The exact cause of inflammatory bowel disease is unclear, but an abnormal immune response occurs. A general principle of IBD is the gut immune system becomes overactive to the normal intestine. In addition, a genetic component seems to be present, especially with Crohn's disease.[25]

Inflammatory bowel disease cannot be diagnosed with a single finding or test. IBD is a clinical syndrome based on symptoms, physical exam, lab, imaging, endoscopy, and biopsy results. Presenting complaints are commonly diarrhea, weight loss, abdominal pain, and occasionally hematochezia. Exam findings can include RLQ tenderness, abdominal distention, and fistula formation. **Extraintestinal** findings include episcleritis, erythema nodosum, pyoderma gangrenosum, aphthous oral ulceration, and joint inflammation (sacroiliitis or symmetric arthritis).

Labs can reveal increased ESR, CRP, and mild anemia. Serologic antibodies linked to Crohn's include anti saccharomyces cerevisiae (ASCA) and linked to ulcerative colitis include anti-neutrophil cytoplasmic antibodies (PANCA). Stool inflammatory markers, stool lactoferrin, and calprotectin can be useful to monitor but are not specific to inflammatory bowel disease. Patients with an elevated PANCA are more likely to have moderate to severe disease.[26] An acute infection can mimic inflammatory bowel disease and is a common contributor to a "flare". Always check stool culture, O+P, and C. diff.

Imaging with CT may reveal intestinal wall inflammation, signs of bowel obstruction, and/or complications like fistula, perforation, or abscess. Enhanced imaging, **CT enterography (CTE)** (use of low-density oral contrast), provides detailed small bowel mucosal images. A similar MRI protocol, MR enterography (MRE), has been valuable in demonstrating the small bowel wall thickening, enhancement of the intestinal wall, and vascularity of the small bowel wall. MRE can be used to evaluate active inflammation vs chronic scarring of the small bowel.[27] However, MRE is very rarely used for inpatient evaluation. Severe ulcerative colitis may have a dilated colon and signs of bowel pneumatosis in severe cases of toxic megacolon.

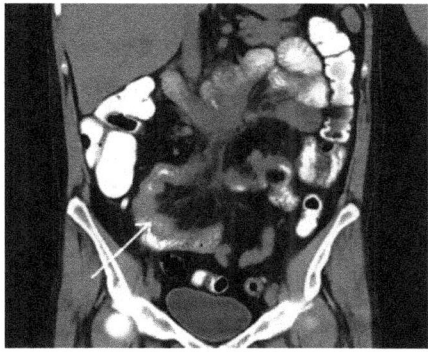
CTE: ileitis

A colonoscopy with an evaluation of the terminal ileum is the main diagnostic test for inflammatory bowel disease. Direct visualization and biopsy sampling are the keys to diagnosis. **Ulcerative colitis** exhibits confluent inflammation extending up from the rectum with erythema, shallow ulceration, and exudate. **Capsule endoscopy** can be used to investigate the small bowel. However, caution is needed since a stricture could lead to capsule retention and the need for surgical resection. Capsule endoscopy is rarely used for inpatient evaluation.

Crohn's disease was first reported in 1932 by Dr. Burrill Crohn documenting patients with regional inflammation of the ileum requiring surgery. Crohn's is a chronic inflammatory condition which can occur in any portion of the digestive tract, but involvement is most common in the ileum and/or colon. Presentation is usually **early in life**, with most diagnosed cases occurring between the ages of 10 and 30. Crohn's is more common in Caucasians, westernized nations, urban environments, and in Jewish heritage.[28] Cigarette smoking can increase the risk of Crohn's.

The inflammation of Crohn's involves the entire wall of the gut **(transmural)**. Chronic inflammation can result in scarring/stenosis and lead to fistula development between the involved bowel and surrounding organs/skin. Involvement of gut mucosa is intermittent **(patchy with skip areas)**. In general, three patterns of Crohn's disease clinical activity exist:

1. Inflammatory Crohn's includes diarrhea, inflammation of gut, and increased CRP, ESR, lactoferrin, calprotectin, and platelets. Abscess is a potential severe complication inflammatory Crohn's.

2. Fibro stenosing Crohn's is a slower form of inflammation. Patients may present with abdominal pain, bowel obstruction (distention, dilated loops of bowel), and minimal acute inflammation.

3. Fistulizing Crohn's is the most aggressive disease with connections between the involved gut and other organs. Fistulas can develop between loops of bowel, bladder, vagina, or skin.

Treatment of inflammation (achieve remission) is the goal of medical therapy for Crohn's disease. Once remission has been achieved, maintenance of remission with other medications is needed. **Active Crohn's** in a hospitalized patient usually requires treatment with oral prednisone or IV solumedrol to induce remission.[29] Dosing of solumedrol over 60 mg IV daily does not confer additional benefit.[30] **Steroids do not maintain remission** and side effects of steroids are well known. After a couple of weeks of steroids, tapering should begin.

5-ASA products are controversial for Crohn's. Data suggest improved remission with colonic Crohn's disease, but not small bowel Crohn's. For mild to moderate Crohn's, 5-ASA products can be considered protective for the colon. Antibiotics are useful for fistulizing or perianal Crohn's disease, where an infectious component may occur as well. In general, antibiotics are unnecessary for mild mucosal inflammatory bowel disease.

Antitumor necrosis factor (anti-TNF) therapies have become the major regimen for severe Crohn's disease. The potent nature of these biologic treatments to suppress acute inflammation helps **induce and maintain remission**. However, immune suppression can result **in the reactivation of latent tuberculosis and hepatitis B** or spur the development of malignancy. Prior to initiating anti-TNF therapies, screen for tuberculosis and hepatitis B, and have a detailed discussion with your patient regarding the risk of infection/malignancy. Anti-TNF medications are rarely started on inpatients. Maintaining remission as an outpatient involves other medications like azathioprine, methotrexate, vedolizumab, mirikizumab, upadacitinib, and anti-TNF therapies. 5-ASA products, steroids including budesonide, and antibiotics do not maintain remission.

Complications of Crohn's are related to stenosis with resulting bowel obstruction and fistulizing disease with the formation of a fistula and/or abscess. Extensive small bowel disease may lead to **B12, vitamins A/E/D/K nutrient deficiencies**. Ileal Crohn's frequently results in bile salt deficiency since bile salts are reabsorbed in the terminal ileum, leading to diarrhea. The malabsorption of fatty acids can lead to **nephrolithiasis** as fatty acids bind calcium, leaving oxalate free to be absorbed and deposited in the kidney.

With colonic involvement in Crohn's, the risk of colorectal cancer is increased. After 8-10 years of Crohn's diagnosis, patients should have a colonoscopy, and repeat colonoscopy every 2 years with biopsies to monitor for signs of dysplasia or colon cancer. Even with excellent medical therapies, 40 to 50% of Crohn's patients will have an operation at some point.

Ulcerative colitis is mucosal inflammation limited to the colon. In contrast to Crohn's, the inflammation pattern is **continuous**. The inflammation starts in the rectum and can extend to the cecum. The symptoms are related to mucosal inflammation and reduced water reabsorption capacity of the colon, resulting in diarrhea.

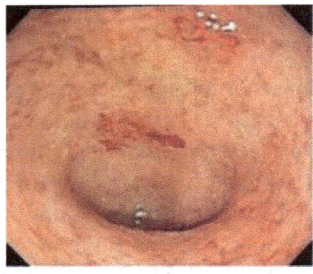
Colonoscopy: ulcerative colitis

The main category of medication for ulcerative colitis is 5-ASA products. 5-ASA may help induce remission and is useful for maintaining remission. In addition, the chronic use of 5-ASA may decrease the lifetime risk of colorectal cancer for ulcerative colitis.[31] 5-ASA products are available in different formulations for release in the small bowel, ileum, or colon with oral use. In addition, 5-ASA suppositories and enemas are available and useful for localized ulcerative colitis.

For acute ulcerative colitis, treatment with oral prednisone or IV solumedrol can be used to induce remission.[32] Dosing of **solumedrol over 60 mg IV daily** is not more effective.[33] In addition, steroid suppositories and enemas are available for localized ulcerative colitis. Antitumor necrosis factor (anti-TNF) therapies are also effective for ulcerative colitis. The potent nature of these biologic treatments in suppressing acute inflammation has been shown to help induce and maintain remission. However, immune suppression could result in the reactivation of latent tuberculosis, hepatitis B, or the development of malignancy.

Prior to initiating anti-TNF therapies, **screening for tuberculosis** with PPD and/or TB spot serology, hepatitis B serologies, and detailed discussion with the patient regarding the risk of infection/malignancy potential should occur.

Cyclosporine is a calcineurin inhibitor and is the last medical option for severe ulcerative colitis. Typically, it is considered after a week of IV steroids with no response. Potential toxicity includes renal dysfunction, infection from immunosuppression, and seizures (especially in patients with hypomagnesemia). With advancements in other medications for inflammatory bowel disease, cyclosporine is rarely (if ever) used, and it is only chosen in hopes of preventing emergent colectomy.

Since ulcerative colitis only involves the colon, surgery with complete removal of the colon can be curative. In severe cases, not responding to medical therapy or in case of suspected dysplasia or cancer, a total proctocolectomy with either an ileostomy or an anal sphincter-sparing operation with an ileoanal pouch anastomosis.

Forms of ulcerative colitis include 1. ulcerative proctitis (limited to the rectum), 2. ulcerative proctosigmoiditis (rectum and sigmoid colon), and 3. pan colitis (involving most of the colon). Complications of ulcerative colitis include severe hematochezia and the formation of toxic megacolon. The colonic wall can become ischemic with extensive inflammation, and perforation can occur. Like Crohn's disease, chronic inflammation with ulcerative colitis increases the risk of colon cancer. After 8-10 years of diagnosis from ulcerative colitis, patients need routine colonoscopy every 2 years with colonic biopsy to evaluate for signs of dysplasia or colon cancer.

Extraintestinal manifestations of ulcerative colitis include primary sclerosing cholangitis, pyoderma gangrenosum, and Sweet syndrome (acute febrile dermatosis). Approximately 25% of ulcerative colitis patients will have surgery.

14. Dysphagia

Take-Aways:

- *Swallowing difficulty can be divided into two categories: oropharyngeal or esophageal.*
- *Divide patient symptoms into either liquid or solid food dysphagia.*
- *Solid food dysphagia suggests a mechanical narrowing of the esophagus.*
- *Acute dysphagia in adults is usually related to a "food bolus." Food bolus is most likely related to meat impaction in a narrowed esophagus.*
- *An EGD is needed to evaluate for mechanical causes and exclude malignancy.*

Swallowing is a complex process involving precise neurologic control of the mouth, oropharynx, and esophagus muscles. Transfer of food from the mouth into the esophagus **(oropharyngeal phase)** is frequently related to neurologic dysfunction. Food movement through the esophagus into the stomach **(esophageal phase)** is usually related to structural/mechanical issues of the esophagus. Rarely inflammation of the esophagus (eosinophilic esophagitis) or esophageal motility disorders can cause esophageal dysphagia. **Odynophagia** is a pain upon swallowing. Most dysphagia complaints are chronic except for acute dysphagia with an object in the esophagus **(typically food bolus).**

With the patient's history, determine the duration, type of foods, and any prior neck surgery or injuries. Weight loss suggests a significant swallowing disorder. A change in voice or speech could indicate a neurologic disorder. Associated symptoms, including GERD, weight loss, or cough while eating, should be evaluated. Finally, classify symptoms into either liquid or solid food dysphagia.

Past medical history of neurologic disorders, tobacco or EtOH use, and previous endoscopies are useful clinical information. On examination, evaluate the neck, lymph nodes, chest, and abdomen. Labs are generally not instructive.

Imaging with a routine chest x-ray and/or CT imaging of the chest can be helpful to exclude mass lesions or extra-luminal compression of the esophagus from a mediastinal structure.

Pathology	Type	Frequency	Association
Schatzki ring	solid	intermittent	belching
Eosinophilic esophagitis	solid	intermittent	asthma
Esophageal cancer	solid	progressive	tobacco
Stroke	liquid	progressive	pneumonia
Parkinson's	both	progressive	pneumonia
Achalasia	both	progressive	weight loss

Schatzki's ring is a narrowing of the lower esophagus in association with a hiatal hernia. The ring is mucosal tissue that causes intermittent difficulty swallowing solid foods. Boston radiologist Richard Schatzki first described it in 1950. Treatment is **endoscopic dilation** of the ring during an EGD. PPI therapy after endoscopic dilation will reduce the risk of reformation of the Schatzki ring.

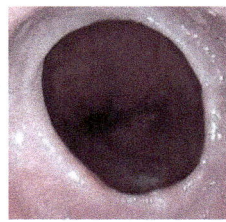 EGD: Schatzki ring

Acute dysphagia related to the impaction of food (food bolus) related to the Schatzki ring commonly occurs. IV glucagon (can lower the pressure of the lower esophageal sphincter) is frequently tried to allow an acute food bolus to pass spontaneously. However, a recent study showed no more effectiveness over a placebo with spontaneous passage of a food bolus.[34] Adverse events of glucagon are rare, so continued use may occur. Other objects (**coins or batteries**) can become "stuck" in the esophagus. Ideally, endoscopic removal occur as soon as possible (within 12 hours).

Eosinophilic esophagitis (EE) is an allergic inflammation of the esophagus characterized by significantly increased eosinophils in the mucosa. Symptoms include **heartburn and intermittent dysphagia**. EE frequently occurs in young males. The exact cause of EE is unknown, but the most prominent theories are related to food and swallowed allergens. EGD will frequently show mucosal rings in the esophagus. Treatment with steroids, proton pump inhibitors, and dietary exclusion diets have been tried. With acute dysphagia, removal of food bolus and gentle dilation of the esophagus with EGD can be performed. The risk of esophageal perforation after dilation is higher with eosinophilic esophagitis.

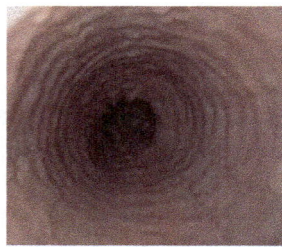 EGD: esophageal rings

Esophageal cancer results in dysphagia from a mechanical narrowing of the esophagus. Solid food becomes progressively difficult to swallow as the tumor grows. Smoking, EtOH intake, and GERD are risk factors. Associated heartburn, weight loss, and chest pain can occur. **Endoscopic evaluation is needed in cases of dysphagia to exclude malignant causes.**

Cerebral vascular accident (stroke) is the most frequent cause of **oropharyngeal dysphagia**. The neurologic control of swallowing is represented in both brain hemispheres. Neurologic control of swallowing becomes impaired with some strokes. Oropharyngeal dysphagia increases the **risk of aspiration pneumonia**. Speech pathology assessment of swallowing and/or a modified barium swallow (radiologic monitoring of swallowed barium) are common after a stroke.

If swallowing deficits are noted, a **gastrostomy tube** is suggested to maintain enteral nutrition and minimize the risk of aspiration. The affected brain area can improve with time, or the unaffected hemisphere can provide compensatory control of swallowing. The oropharyngeal dysphagia from a stroke can improve with time so the **gastrostomy tube is not necessarily permanent**.

Parkinson's disease is a progressive neurological disease that affects the dopamine-producing neurons of the brain. Symptoms of tremor, muscle stiffness, and imbalance can occur. **Oropharyngeal dysphagia is common in Parkinson's**. Symptoms of liquid and solid food dysphagia occur with associated cough and/or aspiration pneumonia. As symptoms progress, oral intake can become impossible, and enteral feeding with a gastrostomy tube may become necessary.

Achalasia is the best-characterized esophageal motility disorder and is caused when normal peristalsis becomes weak and/or absent. In addition, the relaxation of the lower esophageal sphincter of the esophagus becomes disordered. Achalasia is characterized by **liquid dysphagia** with progressive symptoms. Eventually, effortless regurgitation of food/liquids will occur. Food and liquid in the esophagus are suggestive of achalasia. Imaging with a barium swallow **(esophagram)** classically will reveal a dilated esophagus with a narrow lower esophageal sphincter. Formal diagnosis with an esophageal motility study can define achalasia into distinctive subtypes.

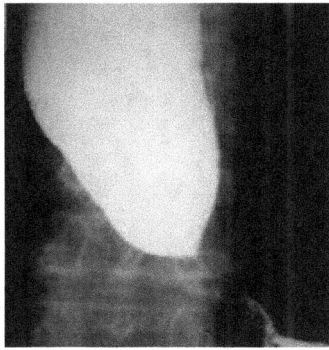
EGD: achalasia

Once diagnosed, outpatient treatment is directed to improve lower esophageal sphincter relaxation. This can be achieved through dilation, Botox injection, or weakening of the lower esophageal sphincter strength by endoscopic or surgical myotomy. Peroral endoscopic myotomy (POEM) is a developing endoscopic technique that is highly effective and can avoid the need for surgery.

15. Nausea/vomiting

Take-Aways:

- *N/V is usually related to an upper digestive disorder.*
- *PUD, pancreatitis, and gallbladder disease are common causes.*
- *Numerous medications can cause or worsen nausea.*
- *When other causes are excluded, gastroparesis should be considered.*
- *Inner ear or intracranial issues are rare causes of nausea/vomiting.*

Nausea is the sensation of needing to vomit and can have associated hypersalivation or dizziness. **Vomiting** is the forceful expelling of gastric contents. Carefully question patient symptoms to differentiate between vomiting and **regurgitation** (passive return of digestive fluids into the mouth). Acute or chronic nausea/vomiting can exist. Vomiting is a complex interaction between the brain and the digestive tract.

The **chemoreceptor trigger zone (CTZ)** in the floor of the fourth ventricle receives afferent stimuli from the GI tract and/or inner ear/vestibular system via neurotransmitters, hormones, and drugs. Vomiting occurs after the CTZ communicates with the vomiting center in the brainstem to produce a response resulting in abdominal muscle contraction, lower esophageal sphincter relaxation, and gastric smooth muscle contraction. Rarely, tumors or intracranial disorders involving the CTZ or vomiting center will cause nausea/vomiting.

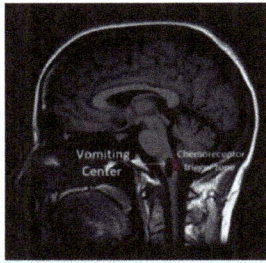

CT: vomiting center / CTZ

Emesis occurs with abdominal wall muscles contracting, relaxation of the lower esophageal sphincter, and contraction of the gastric smooth muscle. When interviewing patients, determine if nausea is **acute** (<4 weeks) or **chronic** (> 4 weeks). Also, ask for any associated symptoms indicating a GI source, like abdominal pain, diarrhea, and weight loss. Symptoms like headache or visual change can indicate an intracranial source of vomiting. Finally, motion sickness, ear ringing, and head position change causing nausea/vomiting could point towards an inner ear/labyrinthine process.

The timing of vomiting after eating is an important clue, especially for issues like gastroparesis. The type of vomitus can be instructive; undigested food points toward an esophageal or gastric issue, while blood makes PUD more likely.
Assess **hydration**. Dehydration can worsen nausea/vomiting. IV fluids will reduce nausea. An abdominal exam and a focused neurologic exam will screen for a potential diagnosis. **Lab testing** will include a CBC, BMP, LFTs, lipase, urinalysis, and urine pregnancy test (age-appropriate females). Significant vomiting can result in hypochloremic hypokalemic **metabolic alkalosis**.

Imaging with **abdomen series and/or CT scan** is useful for acute symptoms. Chronic symptoms can be evaluated by a gastric emptying scan and HIDA scan. In cases of suspected brainstem causes**, an MRI of the brain/brainstem** is needed. EGD is the most helpful to evaluate the esophagus and stomach.

Condition	Duration	Association
Gastroenteritis	acute	diarrhea
Post-operative	acute	inhaled anesthesia
Peptic ulcer (PUD)	acute and chronic	epigastric pain
Medications	acute and chronic	opiates, chemotherapy
Gastroparesis	chronic	weight loss
Cannabis hyperemesis	chronic	relief with hot showers

Viral gastroenteritis or food-borne illness are common causes of acute nausea/vomiting. Rotavirus, norovirus, and staph aureus are common pathogens. IV fluids, supportive care, and antiemetics are useful. Stool studies are needed. Giardia outbreaks can occur in community settings like daycare centers and nursing homes.

Post-operative nausea/vomiting (PONV) can last up to 24 hours after surgery. The combination of anesthetic agents, opioid analgesia, and pain can worsen nausea. **Risk factors for post-op nausea** include female gender, history of motion sickness, and use of volatile anesthetic gas. Dexamethasone and ondansetron are common medications used to reduce PONV.

PUD or gastritis can be caused by H. pylori and NSAID use. Eating typically will worsen nausea when mucosal irritation is present. Bloating, belching, or heartburn can occur. PUD must be excluded if hematemesis is present. For treatment, PPI or H_2 blockers are the most effective medications.

Medications are a frequent contributor to nausea/vomiting. A careful review of the medication list, including OTC and supplements, is needed. Medications that promote the release of dopamine, such as digoxin and opiates, can interact with the chemoreceptor trigger zone. Other medications, such as chemotherapies, antibiotics, and SSRIs, are also known to cause nausea.

Gastroparesis is a slowing of gastric emptying without structural pyloric obstruction. Normally the stomach has 3 peristaltic contractions per minute. A variety of conditions **including diabetes, prior gastric surgery, medications, and neurologic conditions** can change the peristaltic contractions. In addition, poor relaxation of the pylorus may coexist and further slow gastric emptying.

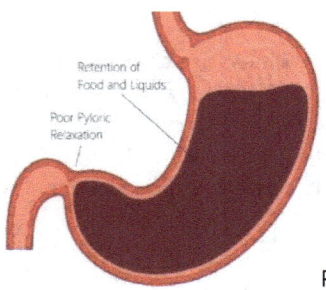

Poor gastric emptying

With food and liquid accumulation in the stomach, nausea, vomiting, weight loss, and upper abdominal bloating develop. Vomitus can contain undigested food eaten many hours or days earlier. An EGD is needed to exclude mechanical blockage of the pylorus. A gastric emptying scan (nuclear medicine imaging) will reveal delayed gastric emptying 4 hours after a standard test meal. Normally, 90% of food eaten will have emptied the stomach after 4 hours. A gastric emptying scan is not routinely done for inpatients.

Gastroparesis treatment is IV hydration, eating small frequent meals that are low fat/low fiber, control of blood sugar, and prokinetic medications. **Metoclopramide** and **domperidone (not FDA-approved)** are the mainstay of treatment. However, using the lowest dose possible of metoclopramide is advised secondary to potentially serious side effects.

Cannabis hyperemesis is an increasing problem with the growing use of marijuana. Patients complain of nausea and vomiting without other underlying causes. Usually, several years of previous marijuana use is noted. A cyclical pattern of intermittent morning nausea for weeks or months precedes significant vomiting with signs of dehydration. A clinical pearl: **Patients often report nausea relief with a warm shower or bath.**

16. Diarrhea

Take-Aways:

- *Acute diarrhea will usually resolve spontaneously.*
- *Dehydration is the most serious complication of diarrhea.*
- *Oral rehydration solution or IV replacement is greatly beneficial to minimize dehydration.*
- *Bloody stool or fever suggests inflammatory diarrhea.*
- *Persistent diarrhea needs endoscopic evaluation.*

Diarrhea is a common issue, and associated dehydration is the main reason for hospitalization. Correction of volume and electrolytes with IV fluids is needed. Fluid constantly passes through the digestive system. Daily, over 10 liters of intestinal fluid enter the jejunum, 1 liter of fluid enters the colon, and only 100 ml of fluid is passed in stool.[35] The diarrhea mechanisms include excessive intestinal fluid production, reduced epithelial absorptive capacity, altered GI motility, and ingestion of poorly absorbed material.

The character, volume, color, and presence of blood are important clues. Again, accurate history is critical. Patients may describe many different stool types as "diarrhea." Dietary intake, sick contacts, and travel history are important. A **large volume** of diarrhea suggests **a small intestinal source**, but a **small volume** with blood suggests a **colonic source**. Fever, night sweats, or bloody diarrhea suggest bacterial or inflammatory diarrhea.

Dehydration is the major complication of diarrhea. Vital signs, mentation, and skin turgor suggest volume status. Examine the abdomen to evaluate for pain or signs of toxicity. Labs include BMP, CBC, stool studies for routine culture, C. Diff, and O+P. Stool WBC or lactoferrin suggest mucosal irritation of the gut. **Hematochezia** warrants an endoscopic exam with a sigmoidoscopy or colonoscopy after IV fluid rehydration.

Causes	Type of Diarrhea	Association
Viral gastroenteritis	watery, large volume	community outbreaks
Bacterial	bloody, small volume	fever, abdominal pain
Food-borne	variable	vomiting
Medications	watery	antibiotics, metformin

Viral gastroenteritis is the most common cause of diarrhea. Infections like rotavirus and norovirus can lead to significant dehydration. Diarrhea is usually watery and has a large volume related to intestinal secretion. Abdominal pain and vomiting can exist. Stool markers of inflammation are usually absent. Community outbreaks can occur due to their highly contagious nature. Daycare centers, cruise ships, and nursing homes experience outbreaks. Fortunately, the infection is usually short-lived and will clear spontaneously in a few days. **Post-infectious inflammatory bowel disease (IBS) is common** for several weeks to months after acute gastroenteritis.

Bacterial causes of diarrhea include excessive intestinal secretion by cholera toxin and inflammatory diarrhea with blood **(dysentery)** from shigella, salmonella, and campylobacter. Bloody stool, abdominal pain, tenesmus, and fever can occur with inflammation. Risk factors for bacterial diarrhea include ongoing PPI use, advanced age, and immunosuppression. Dehydration is the main risk. Antibiotics are the mainstay of treatment. Inflammatory diarrhea can be related to inflammatory bowel disease.

Clostridium difficile (C.diff) is of particular importance for inpatients. C. diff is a bacterial infection that occurs when the stool microbiome becomes unbalanced. Frequently, systemic antibiotics for other infections reduce the healthy bacteria, resulting in excessive growth of C. diff. Elderly or malnourished patients are especially vulnerable. Once, C. diff was just a hospital illness, but now, community cases exist. A thick membrane may develop on the colonic mucosa **(pseudomembranous colitis)** in serious cases.

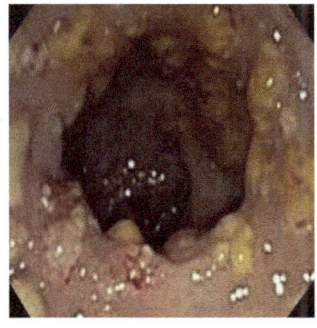 Colonoscopy: pseudomembranes

C. diff can exist as inactive **"spores"** that survive even after successful treatment. Colonization of the colon with C. diff is a risk factor for relapse, especially if another systemic antibiotic is started. C. diff produces two toxins, A and B. For diagnosis, stool **testing for C. diff toxin** is standard. Frequently, testing is performed using polymerase chain reaction (PCR). However, C. diff PCR cannot differentiate between colonization and active infection. Stool testing for **glutamate dehydrogenase antigen** (antibodies to a protein produced by C. diff) is also used to screen for infection.

An acute infection is likely if the stool toxin and GDH are positive. If stool toxin and GDH are negative, active C. diff is unlikely. For indeterminate results, clinical symptoms and/or C.diff **nucleic acid amplification testing (NAAT)** can be used. A sizable number of patients have "colonization" with C. diff but do not have an active infection. **Differentiation between active infection and colonization is important** (and at times exceedingly difficult) since antibiotic treatment is unnecessary for patients with colonization.

Treatment requires patient isolation to minimize the spread of infection and antibiotic treatment for the acute infection. Recent updates from the Infectious Diseases of America Society recommend **fidaxomicin** be considered as the first-line treatment for C. diff. An alternative is **vancomycin**. Both fidaxomicin and vancomycin have low systemic absorption. However, increasing bacterial resistance to vancomycin is a concern. With severe C. diff, rectal vancomycin and/or IV metronidazole can be added.

An advantage of **fidaxomicin** is its reduced effect on the healthy microbiome. To minimize recurrence, a prolonged tapering dose of medication has been suggested after initial treatment. If patients are not responding to antibiotics, a fecal transplant can be considered an experimental treatment. In cases of fulminant infection (sepsis or toxic megacolon), surgical removal of the colon is needed.

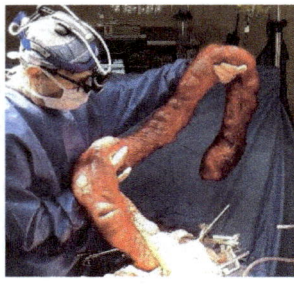
Surgical colectomy

Because C. diff has a high recurrence risk (15-30%), multiple efforts have been made to reduce recurrence after active infection is treated with antibiotics. **Fecal transplantation** has been an investigational treatment with healthy donor stool. However, fecal transplantation has not been standardized, and theoretical risk of infection or other adverse events are risks.

Recently, the Food and Drug Administration (FDA) approved the first standardized commercial fecal transplantation product, Rebyota. Rebyota is prepared healthy stool from qualified donors into a liquid form and is indicated to prevent the reoccurrence of C. Diff after antibiotic clearance of active infection **(not for use in inpatients with active infection)**.

A second FDA-approved product to minimize recurrence is VOWST. VOWST is a bacterial spore suspension from healthy donors placed into capsules for oral patient use. VOWST is not indicated for use with active infection. Finally, another FDA-approved medication, bezlotoxumab, is available to reduce recurrence risk. **Bezlotoxumab** is a human monoclonal antibody for IV infusion that can neutralize C. diff toxin B. Again, bezlotoxumab is not indicated to treat an active C. diff infection.

Parasitic diseases are common causes of diarrhea. Real-time PCR testing for Entamoeba histolytica, giardia lamblia, and Cryptosporidium parvum is available. Giardia is a common parasitic cause of diarrhea. **Risk factors** include travel, hiking, drinking stream water, and daycare centers. **Symptoms** include abdominal pain, nausea, weight loss, and foul-smelling diarrhea. Lactose intolerance will occur in up to 40% of giardia infections and may persist for several months.[36] Stool testing for ova and parasites with routine microscopy is being used less frequently. **PCR stool antigen testing use is increasing.** Treatment of parasitic infections with metronidazole or nitazoxanide is suggested.

Food-borne diarrhea can occur soon after ingesting contaminated food **or** several days later. Ingestion of toxins may result in symptoms of nausea, vomiting, diarrhea, fever, and abdominal pain. **Risk factors** include advanced age, immunosuppression, pregnancy, and chronic PPI use. Severe complications of food-borne diarrhea include hemolytic uremic syndrome with **E.coli (O157:H7 strain),** miscarriages with **listeria**, and symmetric reactive arthritis with **salmonella**. The following table lists the commonly contaminated foods and incubation periods for diarrheal illness.

Pathogen	Foods	Incubation
Bacillus	fried rice/stews	6-12 hours
Staph aureus	meats/potato salad	6-24 hours
Listeria	hot dogs/lunch meat/dairy	1-2 days
E. coli	beef/sprouts	1-2 days
Shigella	seafood/produce	1-2 days
Vibrio	oyster/mussels	1-3 days
Salmonella	dairy/poultry	2-3 days
Campylobacter	meat/poultry	2-3 days

Diarrhea is one of the most common adverse events listed for prescription medications. **Medication-induced diarrhea** is commonly associated with antibiotics, metformin, laxatives, NSAIDs, chemotherapy, colchicine, and PPI therapy. Many over the counter and herbal treatments can lead to diarrhea as well. An accurate medication list and start date for medications is critical for the evaluation of diarrhea.

Increasing immunotherapy/immune checkpoint inhibitors (ipilimumab, pembrolizumab, and nivolumab) for malignancies has increased hospital admissions for diarrhea and/or colitis. If significant diarrhea exists and infectious causes are excluded, a colonoscopy (with colonic biopsies) should be considered to evaluate for immunotherapy-induced colitis. Treatment with prednisone or methylprednisolone is usually effective. Severe or refractory cases may need a biologic infusion with infliximab or vedolizumab.

17. Constipation and Ileus

Take-Aways:

- *Constipation and decreased GI motility are common inpatient symptoms.*
- *Rule out a mechanical obstruction when severe constipation and/or obstipation are present.*
- *Ileus (non-mechanical slowing) is common with pneumonia, pain medications, and surgery.*
- *Abdominal adhesions are the most common cause of complete bowel obstruction.*
- *Colon cancer must be considered with persistent constipation.*

Constipation is common in inpatients due to decreased mobility, pain medication, infection, and recent surgery. Stool softeners and osmotic laxatives like polyethylene glycol are common measures to promote bowel movements. Acute constipation warrants consideration of an undiagnosed obstructive process. Patients may have an ileus or partial small bowel obstruction, which can cause acute constipation. Mechanical obstruction can lead to **dilation and fluid retention** in the small bowel.

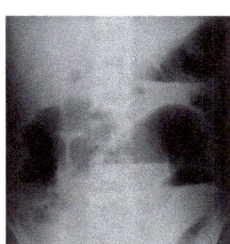 X-ray: ileus

The complaints reported are abdominal pain, distention, and decreased bowel movements. Specific descriptions of the consistency of stool, difficulty in passage (tenesmus/pain), and frequency of bowel movements are needed. Past medical history, including medication use, is important since medications can increase constipation.

The exam includes assessing the thyroid since hypothyroidism can result in constipation. Inspect the abdomen for surgical scars or distention. Bowel sounds become reduced and eventually may become high-pitched with "tinkling" sounds. Severe tenderness is worrisome for impending perforation or peritonitis. A rectal **exam** is mandatory to exclude fecal impaction. Carefully inspect the groin, periumbilical areas, and previous surgical scars for a hernia.

Labs include CBC, BMP, TSH, and calcium. Serum lactate is sometimes ordered when ischemic bowel is suspected. **Hypokalemia** and **hypomagnesemia** are frequently associated with constipation/ileus. Imaging with abdominal x-ray series and/or CT is needed.

Constipation Etiology	Causes	Association
Medication	opioids	post op
Ileus	hypokalemia	pneumonia
SBO	adhesions	Crohn's disease
Colon obstruction	colon cancer	fecal impaction

Medications including opioids, calcium channel blockers, tricyclic antidepressants, oral iron, and anticholinergics are known to cause constipation. Opioid-induced constipation is the most significant risk for inpatients and occurs via activation of the enteric mu-opioid receptors, which reduce gastric, biliary, pancreatic, and intestinal secretions, increase absorption of water from the bowel, and decrease gastric motility.[37]

Medications such as stool softeners, bisacodyl, and polyethylene glycol are useful for mild symptoms. Lubiprostone, a chloride channel activator that increases fluid secretion into the GI tract and peristalsis, can be used for moderate symptoms.

If refractory constipation, exclusion of obstruction with repeat imaging is suggested, and subcutaneous (SC) methylnaltrexone is highly effective in blocking the intestinal effects of opioids. Using fewer opioids and substituting other pain medications like IV acetaminophen after surgery is a strategy to minimize opioid-induced constipation.

Ileus is **nonmechanical slowing of the bowel resulting in** constipation, abdominal bloating, and distention. Ileus is common in hospitalized patients after surgery, with decreased mobility, or with infection. **Pneumonia in an elderly patient** is particularly prone to cause an ileus. Electrolyte disturbances such as **hypokalemia or hypomagnesemia** are also common causes of bowel dysfunction. Treatment is the mobilization of the patient, correction of any electrolyte abnormalities, reducing opioids, and treating the underlying condition (i.e., pneumonia).

A **partial small bowel obstruction (PSBO)** can occur from mechanical causes like adhesions, stricture from previous surgery, Crohn's disease, or a hernia. An accurate surgical history and careful exam of the abdomen for surgical scars/hernias is suggested. Serial abdominal exam and x-ray imaging should be performed to monitor progress.

A nasogastric tube (NG) placement and intermittent wall suction can decompress the stomach and proximal small bowel if significant abdominal symptoms are present. With reduced distention, reduced vomiting and less small bowel dilation will occur. Decreasing small bowel distention is important; increasing distention of the small bowel may cause the vascular supply to become compressed and lead to ischemic changes of the bowel[38]. CT is the most useful imaging modality for finding and monitoring bowel obstruction. If a mechanical "transition point" from a dilated bowel to a diameter bowel is seen, an adhesion is likely the cause of obstruction. Complications like mucosal ischemia, pressure necrosis from adhesions, and perforation can occur. **Surgical consultation** is needed if PSBO is not improving or if a complete SBO is suspected.

Colonic obstruction can occur from colon cancer, fecal impaction, volvulus, or stricture. Historical data like prior diverticulitis, colon surgery, or colonic volvulus may point to the diagnosis. Primary symptoms are abdominal pain and distention. Passage of flatus may stop (obstipation), and a digital rectal exam is needed to exclude a fecal impaction. Bowel sounds may be decreased or absent. CT imaging is the most helpful and can visualize colonic tumors or volvulus.

Volvulus is twisting of bowel around the mesentery and can result in mucosal ischemia and risk of perforation. The sigmoid colon and cecum are the most common locations for a colonic volvulus. Treatment is directed to "untwist" the affected colon. Sigmoidoscopy or colonoscopy is the preferred intervention. With colonoscopy, decompression of the dilated "upstream" colon occurs, and a temporary colonic decompression tube is placed. Once stabilized, surgical consultation is mandatory. Without surgical repair, volvulus will have a high rate of recurrence.

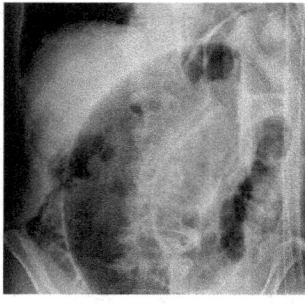
X-ray: colonic volvulus

18. New Mass / Abnormal Imaging

Take-Aways:

- *Increased CT imaging results in the identification of more incidental masses.*
- *Unless the mass is causing symptoms, an outpatient workup is suggested.*
- *Serologic "tumor markers" are NOT diagnostic of cancer.*
- *A tissue biopsy is the key to diagnosis of malignancy.*

With enhanced resolution of CT cross-sectional imaging, the finding of an incidental mass, an "incidentaloma," has become common. Masses may not be malignant but must be evaluated to exclude malignancy. Unless a mass is causing symptoms, an outpatient evaluation after hospital discharge is desirable. However, worrisome symptoms or findings may need hospital evaluation.

Below is a brief review of common digestive malignancies. The workup of a new luminal mass requires endoscopic assessment and occasionally staging with endoscopic ultrasound. The workup of a pancreatic or liver mass requires a tissue diagnosis with biopsy by endoscopic ultrasound or CT-guided biopsy.

Esophageal tumors:

The most common esophageal malignancies are squamous cell carcinoma and adenocarcinoma. Presenting complaints include dysphagia, weight loss, and hematemesis. **Tobacco smoking** and **EtOH** use are risk factors. If CT imaging finds a luminal mass, an upper endoscopy is critical to evaluate and get a tissue biopsy.

Squamous cell carcinoma is usually a proximal tumor in the esophagus and is strongly associated with tobacco use. The **combination of tobacco** and **alcohol** has a strong **synergistic** increase in the risk of malignancy.[39] There is some evidence suggesting a possible causal association between the human papillomavirus **(HPV)** and esophageal squamous-cell carcinoma.[40]

Esophageal adenocarcinoma is usually located in the distal esophagus and is frequently associated with acid reflux, smoking, EtOH, and Barrett's esophagus. **Male predominance** is particularly strong with adenocarcinoma, which occurs about 7 to 10 times more frequently in men.[41]

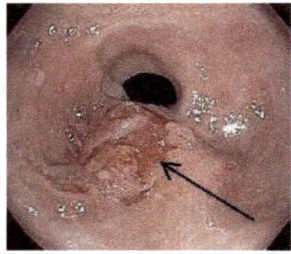 EGD: esophageal adenocarcinoma

Despite being a cause of GERD and a risk factor for gastric cancer, H. pylori seems to be associated with a reduced risk of esophageal adenocarcinoma of as much as 50%.[42] The overall **five-year survival rate** of esophageal cancer in the United States is **around 15%,** with most people dying within the first year of diagnosis.[43]

Submucosal tumors of the esophagus are most commonly benign **leiomyoma**, accounting for roughly two-thirds of all benign tumors.[44] However, **a malignant** gastrointestinal stromal tumor **(GIST)** is also possible. Submucosal tumors are best evaluated with endoscopic ultrasound.

Gastric tumors:

Adenocarcinoma is the most common gastric cancer. The incidence of new gastric cancers has fallen dramatically over the last century. The increase in refrigeration and reduction in salted/preserved foods is believed to be a contributor. **H.pylori** bacteria is **a definite risk factor** for gastric cancer. An enlarged infra-clavicular lymph node on the left side (Virchow's node) or a periumbilical node (Sister Mary Joseph) suggests distant metastatic disease. Any non-healing gastric ulcer should be followed and biopsied to monitor for underlying malignancy.

The stomach is the most common GI location for **lymphoma**. Most gastric lymphomas are diffuse large B-cell type lymphoma (DLBCL) or **mucosa-associated lymphoid tissue lymphoma** (MALT). MALT lymphoma. MALT is strongly associated with H.pylori.

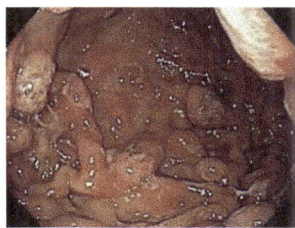 EGD: gastric lymphoma

Submucosal gastric tumors are usually benign gastrointestinal stromal tumors (GIST), commonly arising from the 4th layer of the gastric wall, can grow significantly, and can cause ulceration. **Endoscopic ultrasound** is the most accurate method to evaluate submucosal tumors.

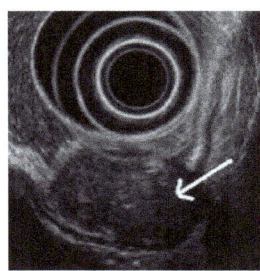 EUS: GIST tumor

Hepatobiliary tumors:

The most common liver tumor is a malignant metastasis from colon cancer. Hepatocellular carcinoma **(HCC),** a malignant transformation of the hepatocytes, is the common primary liver tumor. **Cirrhosis, chronic hepatitis B infection, and hemochromatosis** are risk factors for HCC. Ultrasound, CT scan, and alpha feto-protein (AFP) are screening tools for HCC.

Cholangiocarcinoma is a malignancy of the biliary tract. Risk factors for cholangiocarcinoma are primary sclerosing cholangitis, inflammatory bowel disease, and congenital biliary cysts. Frequently, jaundice will be a presenting symptom related to stenosis (stricture) of the bile duct.

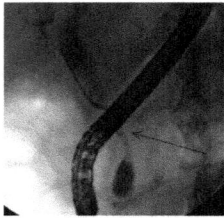 ERCP: bile duct stricture

Pancreatic tumors:

The most common malignancy of the pancreas is adenocarcinoma arising from a pancreatic duct cell. **Pancreatic cancer is the 4th most common cause of cancer death.** Less than 20% of patients will have a resectable tumor after initial diagnosis. Risk factors for pancreatic cancer are a family history of pancreatic cancer, hereditary pancreatitis, and tobacco smoking. **Smoking is estimated to double** the likelihood of **pancreatic cancer** as compared to non-smokers.

Benign pancreatic cysts occur. However, premalignant mucinous pancreatic cysts and malignant intraductal papillary mucinous neoplasms are concerning when a pancreatic cyst is found. Outpatient evaluation and monitoring are needed to exclude a cancerous cyst.

Small bowel tumors:

Small bowel tumors are rare. **Adenocarcinoma** of the small bowel is the most common type of small bowel malignancy and is commonly found in the duodenum or proximal jejunum.

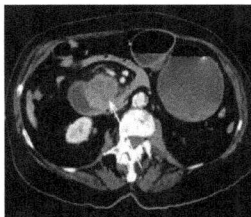 CT: duodenal adenocarcinoma

Chronic inflammatory conditions like **Crohn's or celiac disease** can predispose to malignancy. Carcinoid tumors and intestinal lymphomas rarely occur in the small bowel as well.

Colonic tumors:

Colon cancer is the **2nd leading cause of cancer death in the United States.** The prognosis is linked to the stage at diagnosis. The most common colon malignancy is colonic adenocarcinoma, which develops from a colonic adenoma over time. Colonic tissue transforms to adenoma and later to adenocarcinoma through a series of mutations.[45] The inactivation of adenomatous polyposis coli (APC) mutation occurs early in the progression. Other mutations of tumor suppressor genes (p53) and K-ras proto-oncogene occur as well. The **#1 risk factor** for colorectal cancer is **increasing age**. A personal history of colon polyps, inflammatory bowel disease, and a family history of colon cancer are other risk factors. Rare colon tumor types include carcinoid and lymphoma.

19. Malnutrition / Enteral Tubes

Take-Aways:

- *Basic nutritional assessment begins with a physical exam and BMI.*
- *Enteral nutrition is always preferred. If possible, avoid IV nutrition.*
- *Nasogastric feeding is effective for short-term feeding.*
- *Percutaneous endoscopic gastrostomy (PEG) is the best long-term enteral feeding option.*

Malnutrition is a common condition for hospitalized patients. In general, malnutrition will occur if the intake and absorption of nutrients are insufficient to match the metabolic needs. Weight loss of 20% over time will cause **impaired physiologic bodily functions** (wound healing and immune response).[46] Malnutrition can arise from inadequate intake (cannot afford food, difficulty swallowing, diarrhea/malabsorption) or increased energy expenditure (burns, malignancy, endocrine, or chronic infection) Assessing the patient's normal, highest, and current weight is necessary if malnutrition is suspected. Weight loss can be classified as mild (<5%), moderate (5-10%), or severe (>10%).

Physical exam measures height and weight, examines skin/hair/nails, dentition, dehydration signs, and muscle mass loss. Calculating the BMI is critical. The BMI can estimate metabolic needs.[47]

BMI (kg/m2)	Energy Requirement (kcal/kg/day)
<15	36-45
15-19	31-35
20-29	26-30
>30	15-25

If a patient presents in the hospital with malnutrition, immediate nutritional support should be considered. If a patient is not malnourished on presentation, more reserve exists.

When patients are not eating, the placement of an enteral tube for feeding should be considered. When the expected duration of enteral nutrition **is less than 21 days**, a nasogastric or nasojejunal tube (if post-pyloric feeding is needed) is suggested.

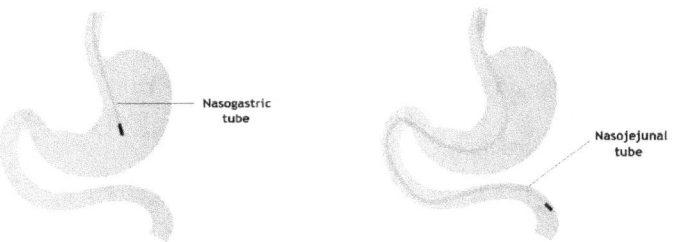

When enteral nutrition is needed for **more than 21 days,** a percutaneous endoscopic gastrostomy tube (PEG) can be placed. If there is a significant risk of aspiration, the PEG can be converted into a percutaneous transgastric jejunal tube **(PEG-J).**

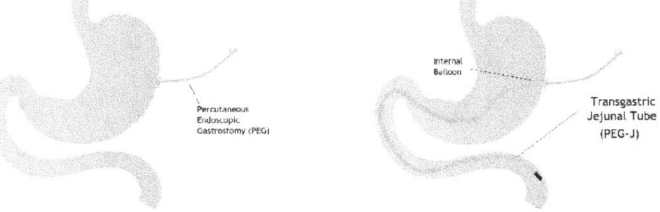

With a tube in place, feeding begins with **bolus** feeding every 4-6 hours with flushing of the tube with free water or **continuous** tube feeding. Patients should remain upright or have the head of bed elevated 30 degrees during bolus feeding and for at least 2 hours after to minimize risk of aspiration.[47]

Gastrostomy tubes should remain in place for at least one month to allow for healing between the gastric and the abdominal wall. An internal bumper on the gastrostomy tube prevents the tube from being dislodged. An external bumper is placed on the tube to prevent internal migration. To minimize the risk of tissue necrosis and infection, the **external bumper should be placed slightly loose** on the skin to allow for rotation of the tube.

At a later time, the initial gastrostomy tube can be changed to a **"replacement"** gastrostomy tube. Replacement tubes have an **internal balloon** instead of a plastic bumper. A replacement gastrostomy tube can be inserted through the established tract into the stomach with the balloon deflated. Then, the internal balloon is inflated to prevent dislodgement.

Parenteral nutrition (IV nutrition) requires a **central venous catheter**, which is prone to infection and reserved for cases of bowel obstruction, short bowel syndrome, or high-output fistulas. It is costly and prone to **complications**. Carefully consider options before starting parenteral nutrition.

20. GI Surgeries

Take-Aways:

- *GI surgeries can lead to abdominal adhesions.*
- *Bariatric surgery alters GI anatomy and can limit endoscopic procedures.*
- *Endoscopy exam via stoma is possible.*

Knowledge of gastrointestinal surgeries will broaden your differential diagnosis. **Previous operations** like appendectomy, groin hernia repair, cholecystectomy, hysterectomy, or intestinal resection can lead to the formation of **adhesions**. Also, complications from recent abdominal surgery can present with abdominal pain.

A Nissen fundoplication is the most common surgical procedure for a hiatal hernia and/or GERD. By wrapping the upper portion of the stomach around itself and suturing it in place, a mechanical barrier is made against the movement of the stomach through the hiatal hernia. The wrap also tightens the lower esophageal sphincter to minimize reflux of gastric contents.

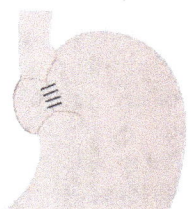

Sleeve gastrectomy is the removal of about 75% of the stomach. Weight loss occurs when patients feel full earlier and eat less. Hormonal changes related to the sense of hunger occur as well. A gastric sleeve is a shorter operation and has fewer complications than a gastric bypass. Importantly for GI endoscopy, the stomach and duodenum are not excluded. Traditional **ERCP and EUS can be performed** in most cases.

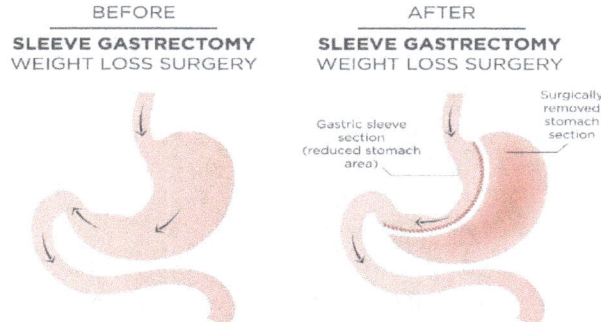

Fistulas occur after a sleeve gastrectomy in **up to 2% of cases**. Fistulas are usually located in the proximal third of the incision line in 89% of cases.[48] Fistulas can be managed with repeat surgery, but endoscopic treatments including clip closure, endoscopic suturing, and internal drainage of fluid collections are developing treatment options.

Roux-en-Y gastric bypass (RYGB) is the most effective surgical technique for weight loss. The upper portion of the stomach is stapled off to create a small pouch and a Y limb of the small intestine is connected to the pouch. The excluded stomach, duodenum, and proximal jejunum are attached to the Y limb. Weight loss occurs with earlier satiety for patients with a much smaller pouch. Malabsorption occurs as the proximal jejunum does not absorb nutrients and the digestive juices from the pancreas and biliary system are not immediately mixing with food to assist digestion. Gut hormones that control hunger and satiety are also changed to reduce appetite. Gastric bypass is a longer operation, takes longer to recover, and with the **exclusion of the proximal upper digestive tract, traditional ERCP or EUS is not possible.**

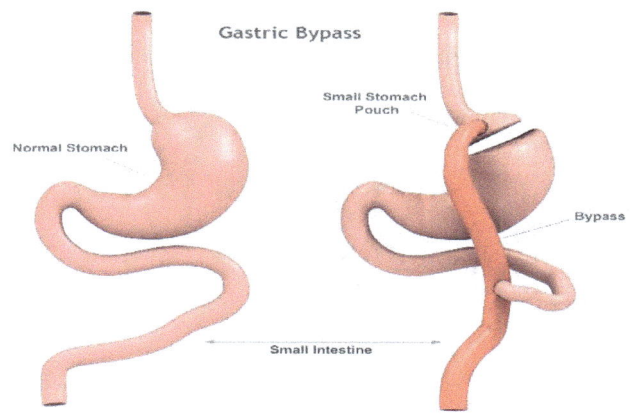

Abdominal pain after RYGB is common. Differential diagnosis includes a **marginal ulcer** at the gastrojejunal anastomosis (up to 15% of patients), gallbladder disease, pseudoobstruction related to an internal hernia or intussusception, **gastric remnant gastropathy from bile reflux**.[47]

Marginal ulceration is characterized by epigastric pain, sometimes "gnawing" which occurs after eating. Since the jejunum does not secrete bicarbonate, the gastrojejunal anastomosis is overly sensitive to gastric acid. Other risk factors for **marginal ulceration** include **tobacco smoking and diabetes**. Treatment for marginal ulceration is PPI therapy. Opening the PPI capsule is preferred to increase absorption and reduce time of ulcer healing.[48] Ursodiol therapy can be useful to alter the composition of bile and help resolve remnant bile gastropathy.[49]

Ileostomy is a connection of the ileum to the abdominal skin. Liquid stool contents come out of the ileostomy into a collection bag. A basic **end ileostomy** results in separation of the ileum from the remaining digestive tract. A temporary **loop ileostomy**, frequently done as a first step in a surgical process, diverts the flow of stool from the remaining digestive tract.

Once the underlying pathology (ulcerative colitis or diverticulitis) heals, the loop ileostomy can be taken down to complete the surgical process. Complications from ileostomy include retraction into the stoma, fistula to the skin near the stoma, stenosis, and a parastomal hernia. Endoscopic exam of the ileum (ileoscopy via stoma) is commonly done to evaluate for bleeding or high ostomy output.

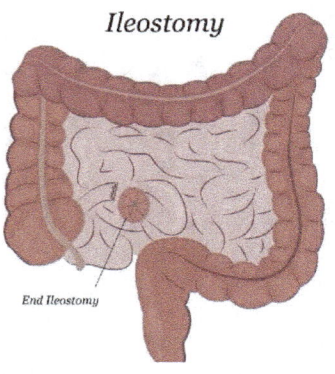

Ileostomy

End Ileostomy

A colostomy is the connection of the colon to the abdominal wall to divert the flow of stool. Passage of stool into a collection bag occurs randomly. The colon distal to the ostomy is bypassed and no stool exits via the anus. A colostomy is frequently placed for **obstructing colon cancer or complicated diverticulitis.** A colostomy with oversewing of the remaning sigmoid colon and rectum, Hartmann's pouch, is commonly done. A repeat operation with reconnection of the colon to the pouch can be done several months later. Complications of a colostomy include bleeding, prolapse of the colon, and parastomal hernia. If lower GI symptoms such as bleeding occur, a colonoscopy via the colostomy can be done after a routine oral bowel preparation.

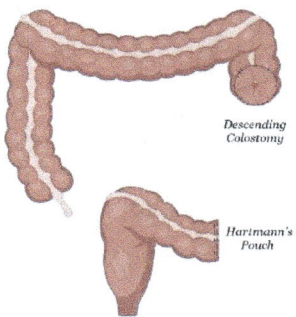

Colostomy with Hartmann's Pouch

Descending Colostomy

Hartmann's Pouch

Ileal pouch anal anastomosis **(IPAA)** involves removal of the colon, stripping of the mucosa from the rectum while preserving the anal sphincters, and attaching a loop of ileum which is folded back on itself in a "J" formation to create a larger reservoir for stool. The larger pouch can hold stool longer and reduce the number of bowel movements.

Pouchitis, an inflammation of the pouch, is a common condition with IPAA. The pouch's mucosa can become inflamed, resulting in diarrhea, mild rectal bleeding, and fecal urgency. Pouchitis may be related to stool alteration since the colonic processing has been removed. Theories of an imbalance of fatty acids are a possible cause of pouchitis. Antibiotics and mesalamine are frequently used for treatment.

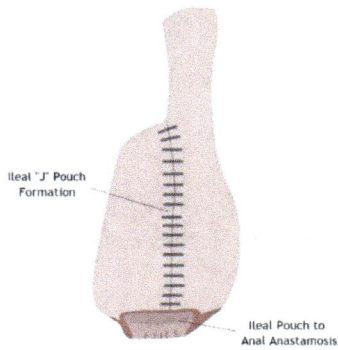

Ileoanal Pouch Anastamosis

Ileal "J" Pouch Formation

Ileal Pouch to Anal Anastamosis

References:
1. McGee S, Abernethy WB III, Simel DL. The rational clinical examination. Is the patient hypovolemic? JAMA 1999; 281: 1022-1029.
2. Agabegi, E, Agagegi, Step up to Medicine, 2008.
3. Falsar, MH, Goldberg E. Acute abdominal pain. Med Clin North Am. 2006; 90:481-503.
4. El-Serag HB, Pandolfino J. Obesity increases oesophageal acid exposure. Gut 2007; 56:749-755
5. Malfertheinner P, Chan F, McColl, K. Peptic ulcer disease. Lancet. 2009; 374: 1449-1461.
6. Everhart J, Khare M, Hill M. Prevalence and ethnic differences in gallbladder disease in the US. Gastro 1999; 117:632-639.
7. Rettenbacher, T, Hollerweger, A. Appendicitis: should diagnostic imaging be performed if the clinical presentation is highly suggestive of the disease? Gastroenterology 2002; 123: 992-998.
8. L. Laine, Upper GI Bleeding ASGE Clinical Update, 2007; 14, 1-4.
9. Parikh, K, Meer, A, Wong, R. Unusual Causes of Upper Gastrointestinal Bleeding. Gastro Endoscopy Clinics. 2015;25:583-605.
10. Wan, D, Sengupta, N. Management of Lower GI bleeding. American Journal of Gastroenterology. 2024; 9:10-14.
11. Khashab, M, Tariq A, Tariq U. Delayed and unsuccessful ERCP are associated with worse outcomes in patients with acute cholangitis. Clin Gastroenterol and Hepatol 2012; 10:1157-61.
12. Tan, M, Schaffalitzky, O, Laursen, S. Association between early ERCP and mortality in patients with acute cholangitis. GIE 2018;87:185-1921.
13. Wiesner et al. Model for end-stage liver disease (MELD) and allocation of donor livers. Gastroenterology (2003) vol. 124 (1) pp. 91-6.
14. Rumack and Matthew. Pediatrics. 1975; 55:871-876
15. Liver complications in Patients with Congestive Heart Failure, Giallourakis C. Gastroenterology Hepatology. 2013 April; 9(4): 244-246.
16. Whitcomb, D. Acute Pancreatitis. NEJM. 2006; 354:2142-2150.

17. Greer J, Thrower E, Yadav D. Epidemiologic and mechanistic associations between smoking and pancreatitis. Curr. Treat Options Gastro. 2015; 13: 332-346.

18. Forsmark C, Baille J; AGA Institute technical review on acute pancreatitis. Gastroenterology.2007;132(5):2022-2044.)

19. Mithofer K, Fernandez-del Castillo C, et al. Acute hypercalcemia causes acute pancreatitis and ectopic trypsinogen activation in the rat.Gastroenterology. 1995;109(1):239.

20. Ranson JH, Rifkind KM, Roses DF, Fink SD, Eng K, Spencer FC (1974). "Prognostic signs and the role of operative management in acute pancreatitis". Surgery, Gynecology & Obstetrics. 139 (1): 69–81

21. Balthazar EJ, Freeny PC, Vansonnenberg E. Imaging and intervention in acute pancreatitis. Radiology. 1994;193 (2): 297-306.

22. Balthazar EJ. Acute pancreatitis: assessment of severity with clinical and CT evaluation. Radiology. 2002;223 (3): 603-13.

23. Ammann RW, Meullhaupt B. The natural history of pain in pancreatitis. 1999;116(5):1132-1140.

24. Bolondi L, Bassi S, Gaiani S, et al. Sonography of chronic pancreatitis. Radio Clinic of North Am.1989; 27(4):815-833.

25. Limbergen V, Russel R, Nimmo E. Genetics of the innate immune response in Inflammatory Bowel Disease. Inflamm Bowel Dis. 2007; 13:338-355.

26. Targan, S, Karp L. Serology and laboratory markers of bowel activity. Inflammatory Bowel Disease. Saunders. 2004:442

27. Griffin N, Grant L, Sanderson J. Small bowel MR enterography. Insights Imaging. 2012; 3:251-263.

28. Podolsky D. Inflammatory Bowel Disease. NEJM. 2002; 347: 417-429.

29. Reference: Lichtenstein G, Cohen R. AGA Position Statement on corticosteroids, immunomodulators, and infliximab in IBD.

30. Turner D, Walsh CM, Steinhart AH, Griffiths AM. Response to corticosteroids in severe ulcerative colitis. Clinical Gastroenterology and Hepatology. 2007;5(1):103-110.

31. Levine, J, Burakoff R. Chemoprophylaxis of colorectal cancer in inflammatory bowel disease. Inflamm Bowel Dis. 2007;13: 1293-1298.

32. Lichtenstein G, Cohen R. AGA Position Statement on corticosteroids, immunomodulators, and infliximab in IBD. Gastroenterology. 2006;130:940-987.

33. Turner D, Walsh CM, Steinhart AH, Griffiths AM. Response to corticosteroids in severe ulcerative colitis. Clinical Gastroenterology and Hepatology. 2007;5(1):103-110.

34. Benito Sanz, M, Tejedor-Tejada, J. Double blind Multicenter randomized clinical trial comparing glucagon vs placebo in the resolution of alimentary esophageal impaction. American Journal of Gastroenterology. 2024;87:119:87-96.

35. Markogiannakis H, Messaris E, et al. Acute mechanical bowel obstruction. World Journal of Gastroenterology. 2007;133(3):432.

36. Camilleri M, Chronic diarrhea: a review on pathophysiology and management. Clin Gastro and Hepatol. 2004;2:198-206.

37. Markogiannakis H, Messaris E, et al. Acute mechanical bowel obstruction. World Journal of Gastroenterology. 2007;133(3):432.

38. Markogiannakis H, Messaris E, et al. Acute mechanical bowel obstruction. World Journal of Gastroenterology. 2007;133(3):432.

39. Prabhu, A; Obi, KO; Rubenstein, JH (June 2014). The synergistic effects of alcohol and tobacco consumption on the risk of esophageal squamous cell carcinoma: a meta-analysis. The American Journal of Gastroenterology. 109 (6): 822–827.

40. Liyanage SS, Rahman B, Ridda I, Newall AT, Tabrizi SN, Garland SM, Segelov E, Seale H, Crowe PJ, Moa A, Macintyre CR (2013). The aetiologic role of human papillomavirus in eosophageal squamous cell carcinoma: a meta-analysis." PLOS ONE. 8 (7): e69238.

41. Rutegård M, Lagergren P, Nordenstedt H, Lagergren J (July 2011). Oesophageal adenocarcinoma: the new epidemic in men? Maturitas. 69 (3): 244–48.

42. Falk, GW (July 2009). "Risk factors for esophageal cancer development." Surgical Oncology Clinics of North America. 18 (3): 469–85.

43. Polednak AP. Trends in survival for both histologic types of esophageal cancer in US surveillance, epidemiology and end results areas. Int. J. Cancer. 2003; 105: (1): 98–100.

44. Lee LS, Singhal S, Brinster CJ, Marshall B, Kochman ML, Kaiser LR, Kucharczuk JC. Current management of esophageal leiomyoma. J Am Coll Surg. 2004;198:136–146.

45. Vogelstein B, Fearon E, Hamilton, S. Genetic alterations during colorectal-tumor development. NEJM. 1998;319:525-532.

46. Klein, S. A primer of nutritional support for gastroenterologists.

47. Metabolic needs can be estimated by the BMI.

48. Aurora, A, Khaitan, L, Saber, A. Sleeve gastrectomy and the risk of leak. Surg Endoscopy. 2012;26:1509-15.

49. Azagury, D, Abu Dayyeh, B Greenwalt, I. Marginal ulceration after Roux-en-Y gastric bypass surgery: Characteristics, risk factors, treatment, and outcomes. Endoscopy 2011;43:950-4.

47. Schulman, A, Chan W, Devery, A. Opened proton pump inhibitor capsules reduce time to healing for marginal ulceration following Roux-en-Y gastric bypass. Clin Gastroenterology Hepatol 2016;15:494-500.

48. Kumar, N, Thompson, C. Ursodiol is effective for treatment of abdominal pain associated with gastritis of the remnant stomach in Roux-en-Y gastric bypass patients. Gastroenterology 2013; 144:s-270.

www.ingramcontent.com/pod-product-compliance
Lightning Source LLC
Chambersburg PA
CBHW071835210526
45479CB00001B/143